Health Promotion in Children and Adolescents through Sport and Physical Activities

Health Promotion in Children and Adolescents through Sport and Physical Activities

Special Issue Editor

Antonino Bianco

MDPI • Basel • Beijing • Wuhan • Barcelona • Belgrade

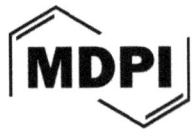

Special Issue Editor
Antonino Bianco
University of Palermo
Italy

Editorial Office
MDPI
St. Alban-Anlage 66
4052 Basel, Switzerland

This is a reprint of articles from the Special Issue published online in the open access journal *Journal of Functional Morphology and Kinesiology* (ISSN 2411-5142) from 2017 to 2019 (available at: https://www.mdpi.com/journal/jfmk/special_issues/adolescents_sport)

For citation purposes, cite each article independently as indicated on the article page online and as indicated below:

LastName, A.A.; LastName, B.B.; LastName, C.C. Article Title. *Journal Name* **Year**, *Article Number, Page Range.*

ISBN 978-3-03897-886-2 (Pbk)
ISBN 978-3-03897-887-9 (PDF)

Contents

About the Special Issue Editor

Antonino Bianco has been assistant professor at the University of Palermo since December 2008. He is also a dean delegate for international programs, a co-founder of the International Ph.D. Program in Health Promotion and Cognitive Sciences, a coordinator and lecturer of the strength and conditioning programs for BSc and MSc courses, a lecturer of exercise physiology courses, and a lecturer of exercise training methodology courses. He has co-authored more than 100 peer-reviewed articles, spoken at more than 30 international events, and co-authored the GSSI Sports Nutrition Award-winning project at ECSS 2017 ("Effects of Ten Months of Intermittent Fasting on Strength, Body Composition, and Metabolism in Athletes"). His main research interests include the following: (1) pediatric exercise and cognitive functions development; (2) the fundamentals of training methodology for muscle hypertrophy; and (3) muscle power, force ratio, and applied biomechanics.

Preface to "Health Promotion in Children and Adolescents through Sport and Physical Activities"

This Special Issue entitled "Health Promotion in Children and Adolescents through Sport and Physical Activities" was developed after I received an interesting phone call from Giuseppe Musumeci, a friend and colleague who, in my opinion, is brilliantly driving JFMK to success. Giuseppe motivated me to manage a Special Issue (SI), and after a short interaction with him and some personal study, I decided to address the topic of this SI to the area mentioned above. Although the title of this SI may seem a bit broad, since the beginning, my intention has been clear: to try to collect more information about the impact that human movement has on the physical and psychological conditions of subjects during all stages of development, also known as the pediatric age. I admit I was surprised when submissions started rolling in. There were many exciting works (unfortunately, we had to reject a few of them for a variety of reasons), and in the end we collected 13 contributions in a short period. In brief, I will present here the core message that this SI book aims to share with the readers. The first part of the book contains three interesting editorials that fit perfectly with the SI's purposes. Sarah West et al. point out the importance of "research that longitudinally assesses how lifelong physical activity [] contributes to life expectancy and mortality", while Ambra Gentile presents an interesting project supported by the European Commission addressing sports and human movement as valid methods of preventing violence and social exclusion. The third editorial by Marianna Alesi et al. also report on a European initiative concerning cognitive and motivational monitoring during enriched sports activities. Interestingly, these three articles have many common points, and the central role of human movement is the driving factor. Among the subsequent contributions, readers will find an interesting review by Riggs Klika et al., in which the terms cancer, pediatric age, and exercise have been properly investigated and presented. Laura Kabiri et al. present data that support the importance of being active at a young age, while Ryan D. Burn and You Fu investigated the interrelationships among motor competence and health-related variables during the pediatric age. The matter of motor competence is addressed by Charlotte JH Hall et al., who suggest that good motor competence is an important correlate of children meeting physical activity guidelines for health. In an original investigation, Yolanda Demetriu et al. provide first insights into how a sports-oriented school can promote students' physical literacy and optimal cognitive performance. Cain CT Clark et al. investigated motor skills in children and highlighted the importance of gender differences, while the work of Michael PR Sheldrick et al. report that sufficient MVPA and excessive screen time were associated with healthy and unhealthy factors, respectively, with relationships sometimes differing by sex. Ewan Thomas and Antonio Palma report that it is possible to consider age-related performance measures to develop exercise interventions that follow the growth characteristics of schoolchildren, while Francisco Tavares et al., in their original investigation, encourage the development of power capacities in the late youth phase when preparing athletes for the senior competition level. Now, at the end of this journey through all the scientific contributions that I had the honor of managing, I want to say thank you to all the lovely people at the MDPI Editorial Office. I felt supported and encouraged to be creative and productive, and I will definitely request a second edition of this successful and interesting Special Issue.

Antonino Bianco
Special Issue Editor

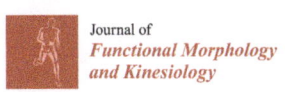

Journal of
*Functional Morphology
and Kinesiology*

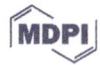

Editorial

The Epidemic of Obesity and Poor Physical Activity Participation: Will We Ever See a Change?

Sarah L. West [1,2,*], Jessica Caterini [2,3], Laura Banks [3] and Greg D. Wells [2]

1   Department of Biology, Trent/Fleming School of Nursing, Trent University, LHS, D231, 1600 West Bank Drive, Peterborough, ON K9L 0G2, Canada
2   Translational Medicine, The Hospital for Sick Children, Toronto, ON M5G 1X8, Canada; jessica.caterini@sickkids.ca (J.C.); greg.wells@sickkids.ca (G.D.W.)
3   Faculty of Kinesiology and Physical Education, University of Toronto, Toronto, ON M5S 2W6, Canada; laura.banks@utoronto.ca
*   Correspondence: sarahwest@trentu.ca or sarahwest@sickkids.ca; Tel.: +1-705-748-1011 (ext. 6129)

Received: 18 May 2018; Accepted: 4 June 2018; Published: 10 June 2018

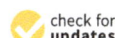
check for
updates

Keywords: obesity; physical activity; adults; children; life expectancy; mortality

---

Obesity is a global epidemic, and researchers have been examining its prevalence and impact for decades [1]. In 2016, The World Health Organization (WHO) estimated that more than 1.9 billion adults over the age of 18 were overweight, and 650 million of these adults were obese [2]. Worldwide obesity in adults has greatly increased in the last ~40 years [2]; a systematic review of over 1700 research studies found that the global proportion of overweight/obese adults increased from 28.8% to 36.9% in males, and 29.8% to 38% in females between 1980 and 2013 [1]. Furthermore, global obesity rates are projected to continue to steadily increase [3].

Unfortunately, the epidemic of obesity is not limited to adults; children and adolescents are overweight and obese at alarming levels worldwide, with many countries reporting prevalence rates of ~20–35% [4–11]. As seen in adults, the proportion of overweight/obese youth continues to rise [1,12]. Even more concerning is that obesity is becoming a prevalent issue in very young children; the WHO estimates that as of 2016, 41 million children under the age of five are overweight or obese [2]. In one a study of over 2000 four-year-old children from Spain, the prevalence of obesity increased from 5.4% to 10.1% over a two-year follow-up [4]. Obesity during childhood/adolescence drastically increases the probability of obesity in adulthood [13,14]. Early-onset obesity is setting children up for a lifelong risk of obesity-associated complications, as it is now understood that early markers of adult cardiovascular disease begin in childhood [15].

Obesity is associated with disorders of almost every system in the body [16]. For example, adults with obesity have increased incidence of cardiovascular disease, diabetes, high cholesterol, and hypertension [17–19]. Childhood obesity is also associated with hypertension, insulin resistance, and liver disease, among others [16]. In a large cohort study of over 8500 nine-year-old Irish children, a staggering 11.1% of the population reported having a chronic illness that impaired daily living [20]. Children who reported living with chronic diseases were more often overweight or obese (32% prevalence) [20]. The negative health effects associated with obesity are not limited to physical outcomes; cognitive function is also decreased in obese children [21,22]. For example, a recent study examined the association of adiposity with achievement and cognitive function in obese children aged 7–9 years old vs. normal-weight children [23]. Compared to normal-weight children, children who were obese had lower performance on tests of reading and math. In the obese children, higher visceral adipose tissue was associated with poorer intellectual abilities and cognitive performance [23]. Published data indicate that an increasing number of children are at risk of obesity-associated physical and cognitive dysfunction, as well as poor psychosocial health (i.e., anxiety, depression) [24], underscoring the need to address this epidemic.

Physical activity is an important, modifiable lifestyle factor that can help improve health outcomes in adults and children, including reducing obesity [25–27], cardiovascular disease [28,29], and diabetes [27,30]. Current WHO global recommendations for physical activity suggest that adults aged 18–64 years of age should engage in at least 150 min of moderate–vigorous physical activity per week, in bouts of at least 10 min of duration [31], and that children aged 5–17 years old should be accumulating 60 min of daily moderate–vigorous intensity physical activity. The WHO report indicates a dose-response relationship with greater physical activity levels associated with additional health benefits in adults and children [31].

Unfortunately, and perhaps not surprisingly, both adults and children are not meeting these physical activity guidelines globally [32–36]. Canadian Health Measures Survey data (2007–2009) indicate that only 15% of Canadian adults are accumulating the recommended 150 min of moderate–vigorous physical activity per week [32], and of them, only 5% accumulate 150 min per week in at least 30-min bouts five or more days per week [32]. According to the Centers for Disease Control and Prevention (CDC) in the United States, only 20.5% of adults in 2015 were meeting the WHO-recommended physical activity guidelines [33]. In an international study of 20 countries, the percentage of adults who reported being physically inactive (sedentary) was between 6.9% (China) and 42.3% (Taiwan) [36].

Children are also not achieving physical activity guidelines; the WHO estimates that globally, 81% of school-aged children are not meeting guidelines of 60 min of physical activity per day [37]. The new Canadian 24-h Movement Guidelines for the Early Years (0–4 years) suggest that preschoolers should engage in at least 180 min per day of physical activities, 60 min of which should be moderate to vigorous daily physical activity [38]. Chaput et al. reported that 38.2% of Canadian preschool children (mean age 3.5 years) were not meeting these physical activity recommendations [39]. When the Canadian 24-h Movement Guidelines were examined in an international sample of over 6000 children, the global prevalence of meeting the recommendations was only 7% [40]. Therefore, the problem of physical inactivity is evident at a very early age.

The information regarding poor physical activity participation, combined with the high prevalence of obesity, is more than just disappointing; it is concerning. There have been no major, successful population intervention strategies to reduce obesity, and there have been no national successes in reducing the burden of obesity in the past 33 years [1]. We know that physical activity is a potent 'medicine' against obesity, yet despite the prominent health benefits of physical activity, participation rates in both adults and children remain low. We are observing a disconnect between the known benefits of physical activity and the number of individuals who actively engage in the recommended amounts. We wonder then, "What kind of data will it take for the general population to decide that physical activity is a necessity to include in their daily lives?" One emerging area of research is examining the association between physical activity and mortality. Perhaps identifying a link between physical inactivity and increased mortality will be the convincing data needed to encourage adherence to physical activity guidelines.

A recent study titled "Impact of healthy lifestyle factors on life expectancies in the U.S. population" by Li and colleagues was published in the prominent American Heart Association journal, *Circulation* [41]. This was a comprehensive, large-scale analysis of how lifestyle factors impact life expectancy in the U.S. population [41]. The authors examined the association of lifestyle-related low-risk factors (specifically: diet, smoking, physical activity, alcohol consumption, and body mass index) using well-collected cohort data including the Nurses' Health Study (NHS), and the Health Professionals Follow-up Study (HPFS). They also used data from the National Health and Nutrition and Examination Surveys (NHANES) to determine the distribution of the lifestyle related factors in the U.S. population, and they derived death rates from the Centers for Disease Control and Prevention

Wide-Ranging Online Data for Epidemiological Research database. At baseline, the authors included 78,865 females and 44,354 males for analysis [41].

Li et al. defined five low-risk factors (diet, smoking, physical activity, alcohol consumption, and body mass index) and examined their impact together and independently on mortality [41]. We will focus on discussing the physical activity findings. Physical activity was measured using a validated questionnaire (updated every two years), and was considered to be a low-risk lifestyle factor if individuals engaged in >30 min per day of moderate or vigorous activity (including brisk walking). To determine how lifestyle factors affected mortality risk, Li et al. calculated the average physical activity level using the last two repeated measurements relative to a mortality event. For example, if a mortality case occurred in 1982–1984, the average of the 1980 and 1982 physical activity questionnaire for that individual was used [41].

Women had a median study follow-up of 33.9 years, and men had a follow-up of 27.2 years. During this time 42,167 deaths were recorded [41]. The authors found that each of the five healthy lifestyle components was significantly associated with the risk of all-cause mortality. A higher dose of physical activity was associated with a decrease in all-cause mortality, death due to cancer, and death due to cardiovascular disease. Specifically, completing 0.1–0.9 h/week of physical activity was associated with a hazard radio (HR) of 0.65 (95% confidence intervals (CI): 0.63–0.66); 1.0–3.4 h/week was associated with a HR of 0.56 (95% CI: 0.54–0.58); 3.5–5.9 h/week was associated with a HR of 5.0 (95% CI: 0.48–0.52); and $\geq$6 h/week was associated with a HR of 0.44 (95% CI: 0.43–0.46) for all-cause mortality [41]. In other words, engaging in physical activity for as little as 0.1 hour/week up to $\geq$6 h/week was associated with a 35–56% reduced risk of death over the follow-up period [41]. The authors estimated gained life expectancy, and found that increased participation in physical activity compared to the most sedentary group was associated with a longer life expectancy [41]. The conclusions from this large and well-designed analysis are clear; modifiable lifestyle factors such as physical activity can improve life expectancy in U.S. adults [41].

Therefore, we return to our previous question, "what kind of data will it take for the general population to decide that physical activity is a necessity to include in their daily lives?" It is evident from Li et al.'s comprehensive study that life expectancy is directly linked with physical activity participation in adults [41]. Will this be the convincing piece of evidence required to convince adults that physical activity participation is necessary? It is unlikely that the results from Li and colleagues' study will lead to large-scale physical activity participation change, because there have been previous studies that also report an inverse, independent association between volume of physical activity and mortality in adults [42–45].

However, let us say, optimistically, that Li et al.'s study does result in knowledge translation and encourages adults to become more physically active to prolong life; do the results also encourage physical activity participation in children? As previously mentioned, Li et al. quantified cumulative average levels of physical activity using the last two repeated measures (i.e., four years) prior to mortality; and therefore they reported that relatively short-term physical activity participation is associated with prolonged life [41]. This may suggest that a long-term sedentary lifestyle during childhood and early adulthood is not problematic. However, we know that this is untrue based on studies that show childhood/lifetime physical activity participation is predictive of physical activity habits, fitness, and cardiovascular health later in life [46,47]. Healthy, active kids often equate to healthy, active adults. Furthermore, the body mass index of children is significantly and positively associated with a family history of obesity [48]; encouraging healthy-weight children leads to healthy-weight adults, which in turn results in the next generation of healthy-weight children.

While the conclusions by Li et al. are important and should not be diminished [41], we are still in need of research that longitudinally assesses how lifelong physical activity, beginning in childhood, contributes to life expectancy and mortality. We acknowledge that this would be a large, expensive, and difficult endeavour given the extensive follow-up it would require, and is likely why this type of study does not yet exist. However, consider the large economic burden of obesity, which has been estimated at $2.0 trillion dollars globally [49]; if we funnelled even a small portion of this money into research, a long-term physical activity and life-expectancy study beginning in childhood is suddenly realistic. We desperately need to change our future obesity outlook; it is our duty as researchers and academics to prioritize future studies that may, in turn, result in the information necessary to trigger large-scale changes in physical activity participation and obesity.

References

1. Ng, M.; Fleming, T.; Robinson, M.; Thomson, B.; Graetz, N.; Margono, C.; Mullany, E.C.; Biryukov, S.; Abbafati, C.; Abera, S.F.; et al. Global, regional and national prevalence of overweight and obesity in children and adults 1980–2013: A systematic analysis. *Lancet* **2014**, *384*, 766–781. [CrossRef]
2. World Health Organization. Obesity and Overweight. 2017. Available online: http://www.who.int/en/news-room/fact-sheets/detail/obesity-and-overweight (accessed on 10 May 2018).
3. The Organisation for Economic Co-operation and Development. Obesity Update 2017. Available online: https://www.oecd.org/els/health-systems/Obesity-Update-2017.pdf (accessed on 10 May 2018).
4. Ortiz-Marron, H.; Ortiz-Pinto, M.A.; Cuadrado-Gamarra, J.I.; Esteban-Vasallo, M.; Cortes-Rico, O.; Rey-Gayo, L.; Ordobas, M.; Galan, I. Persistence and variation in overweight and obesity among the pre-school population of the Community of Madrid after 2 years of follow-up. The eloin cohort. *Rev. Esp. Cardiol.* **2018**. [CrossRef] [PubMed]
5. Sjoberg, A.; Moraeus, L.; Yngve, A.; Poortvliet, E.; Al-Ansari, U.; Lissner, L. Overweight and obesity in a representative sample of schoolchildren—Exploring the urban-rural gradient in Sweden. *Obes. Rev.* **2011**, *12*, 305–314. [CrossRef] [PubMed]
6. Liu, J.M.; Ye, R.; Li, S.; Ren, A.; Li, Z.; Liu, Y.; Li, Z. Prevalence of overweight/obesity in Chinese children. *Arch. Med. Res.* **2007**, *38*, 882–886. [CrossRef] [PubMed]
7. Bertoncello, C.; Cazzaro, R.; Ferraresso, A.; Mazzer, R.; Moretti, G. Prevalence of overweight and obesity among school-aged children in urban, rural and mountain areas of the Veneto Region, Italy. *Public Health Nutr.* **2008**, *11*, 887–890. [CrossRef] [PubMed]
8. Malik, M.; Bakir, A. Prevalence of overweight and obesity among children in the United Arab Emirates. *Obes. Rev.* **2007**, *8*, 15–20. [CrossRef] [PubMed]
9. Hassapidou, M.; Daskalou, E.; Tsofliou, F.; Tziomalos, K.; Paschaleri, A.; Pagkalos, I.; Tzotzas, T. Prevalence of overweight and obesity in preschool children in Thessaloniki, Greece. *Hormones* **2015**, *14*, 615–622. [CrossRef] [PubMed]
10. Kulaga, Z.; Gurzkowska, B.; Grajda, A.; Wojtylo, M.; Gozdz, M.; Litwin, M. The prevalence of overweight and obesity among Polish pre-school-aged children. *Dev. Period Med.* **2016**, *20*, 143–149. [PubMed]
11. Statistics Canada. Body Mass Index of Children and Youth, 2012–2013. 2013. Available online: https://www.statcan.gc.ca/pub/82-625-x/2014001/article/14105-eng.htm (accessed on 10 May 2018).
12. Statistics Canada. Overweight and Obese Youth (Self-Reported). 2014. Available online: https://www.statcan.gc.ca/pub/82-625-x/2015001/article/14186-eng.htm (accessed on 10 May 2018).
13. Whitaker, R.C.; Wright, J.A.; Pepe, M.S.; Seidel, K.D.; Dietz, W.H. Predicting obesity in young adulthood from childhood and parental obesity. *N. Engl. J. Med.* **1997**, *337*, 869–873. [CrossRef] [PubMed]
14. Guo, S.S.; Wu, W.; Chumlea, W.C.; Roche, A.F. Predicting overweight and obesity in adulthood from body mass index values in childhood and adolescence. *Am. J. Clin. Nutr.* **2002**, *76*, 653–658. [CrossRef] [PubMed]
15. Li, S.; Chen, W.; Srinivasan, S.R.; Bond, M.G.; Tang, R.; Urbina, E.M.; Berenson, G.S. Childhood cardiovascular risk factors and carotid vascular changes in adulthood: The Bogalusa Heart Study. *JAMA* **2003**, *290*, 2271–2276. [CrossRef] [PubMed]
16. Gungor, N.K. Overweight and obesity in children and adolescents. *J. Clin. Res. Pediatr. Endocrinol.* **2014**, *6*, 129–143. [CrossRef] [PubMed]
17. Ghandehari, H.; Le, V.; Kamal-Bahl, S.; Bassin, S.L.; Wong, N.D. Abdominal obesity and the spectrum of global cardiometabolic risks in US adults. *Int. J. Obes.* **2009**, *33*, 239–248. [CrossRef] [PubMed]
18. Hu, F.B. Globalization of diabetes: The role of diet, lifestyle, and genes. *Diabetes Care* **2011**, *34*, 1249–1257. [CrossRef] [PubMed]

19. Schulze, M.B.; Hu, F.B. Primary prevention of diabetes: What can be done and how much can be prevented? *Annu. Rev. Public Health* **2005**, *26*, 445–467. [CrossRef] [PubMed]
20. Fitzgerald, M.P.; Hennigan, K.; O'Gorman, C.S.; McCarron, L. Obesity, diet and lifestyle in 9-year-old children with parentally reported chronic diseases: Findings from the growing up in Ireland longitudinal child cohort study. *Ir. J. Med. Sci.* **2018**. [CrossRef] [PubMed]
21. Kamijo, K.; Khan, N.A.; Pontifex, M.B.; Scudder, M.R.; Drollette, E.S.; Raine, L.B.; Evans, E.M.; Castelli, D.M.; Hillman, C.H. The relation of adiposity to cognitive control and scholastic achievement in preadolescent children. *Obesity* **2012**, *20*, 2406–2411. [CrossRef] [PubMed]
22. Chojnacki, M.R.; Raine, L.B.; Drollette, E.S.; Scudder, M.R.; Kramer, A.F.; Hillman, C.H.; Khan, N.A. The negative influence of adiposity extends to intraindividual variability in cognitive control among preadolescent children. *Obesity* **2018**, *26*, 405–411. [CrossRef] [PubMed]
23. Raine, L.; Drollette, E.; Kao, S.C.; Westfall, D.; Chaddock-Heyman, L.; Kramer, A.F.; Khan, N.; Hillman, C. The associations between adiposity, cognitive function, and achievement in children. *Med. Sci. Sports Exerc.* **2018**. [CrossRef] [PubMed]
24. Sagar, R.; Gupta, T. Psychological aspects of obesity in children and adolescents. *Indian J. Pediatr.* **2017**. [CrossRef] [PubMed]
25. Katzmarzyk, P.T.; Barreira, T.V.; Broyles, S.T.; Champagne, C.M.; Chaput, J.P.; Fogelholm, M.; Hu, G.; Johnson, W.D.; Kuriyan, R.; Kurpad, A.; et al. Physical activity, sedentary time, and obesity in an international sample of children. *Med. Sci. Sports Exerc.* **2015**, *47*, 2062–2069. [CrossRef] [PubMed]
26. Ohkawara, K.; Tanaka, S.; Miyachi, M.; Ishikawa-Takata, K.; Tabata, I. A dose-response relation between aerobic exercise and visceral fat reduction: Systematic review of clinical trials. *Int. J. Obes.* **2007**, *31*, 1786–1797. [CrossRef] [PubMed]
27. Fedewa, M.V.; Gist, N.H.; Evans, E.M.; Dishman, R.K. Exercise and insulin resistance in youth: A meta-analysis. *Pediatrics* **2014**, *133*, e163–e174. [CrossRef] [PubMed]
28. Kohl, H.W., 3rd. Physical activity and cardiovascular disease: Evidence for a dose response. *Med. Sci. Sports Exerc.* **2001**, *33*, S472–S483. [CrossRef] [PubMed]
29. Ingul, C.B.; Tjonna, A.E.; Stolen, T.O.; Stoylen, A.; Wisloff, U. Impaired cardiac function among obese adolescents: Effect of aerobic interval training. *Arch. Pediatr. Adolesc. Med.* **2010**, *164*, 852–859. [CrossRef] [PubMed]
30. Eriksson, J.G. Exercise and the treatment of type 2 diabetes mellitus. An update. *Sports Med.* **1999**, *27*, 381–391. [CrossRef] [PubMed]
31. World Health Organization. Global Recommendations on Physical Activity for Health. 2010. Available online: http://apps.who.int/iris/bitstream/handle/10665/44399/9789241599979_eng.pdf;jsessionid=8967C56AE594AB4936F7DD184F2C52A6?sequence=1 (accessed on 10 May 2018).
32. Colley, R.C.; Garriguet, D.; Janssen, I.; Craig, C.L.; Clarke, J.; Tremblay, M.S. Physical activity of Canadian adults: Accelerometer results from the 2007 to 2009 Canadian health measures survey. *Health Rep.* **2011**, *22*, 7–14. [PubMed]
33. Centre for Disease Control and Prevention. Nutrition, Physical Activity, and Obesity: Data, Trends and Maps. Available online: https://nccd.cdc.gov/dnpao_dtm/rdPage.aspx?rdReport=DNPAO_DTM.ExploreByLocation&rdRequestForwarding=Form (accessed on 10 May 2018).
34. Ranasinghe, C.D.; Ranasinghe, P.; Jayawardena, R.; Misra, A. Physical activity patterns among South-Asian adults: A systematic review. *Int. J. Behav. Nutr. Phys. Act.* **2013**, *10*, 116. [CrossRef] [PubMed]
35. Marsaux, C.F.; Celis-Morales, C.; Hoonhout, J.; Claassen, A.; Goris, A.; Forster, H.; Fallaize, R.; Macready, A.L.; Navas-Carretero, S.; Kolossa, S.; et al. Objectively measured physical activity in European adults: Cross-sectional findings from the Food4Me Study. *PLoS ONE* **2016**, *11*, e0150902. [CrossRef] [PubMed]
36. Bauman, A.; Bull, F.; Chey, T.; Craig, C.L.; Ainsworth, B.E.; Sallis, J.F.; Bowles, H.R.; Hagstromer, M.; Sjostrom, M.; Pratt, M. The international prevalence study on physical activity: Results from 20 countries. *Int. J. Behav. Nutr. Phys. Act.* **2009**, *6*, 21. [CrossRef] [PubMed]
37. World Health Organization. 10 Facts on Physical Activity. 2017. Available online: http://www.who.int/features/factfiles/physical_activity/en/ (accessed on 10 May 2018).

38. Tremblay, M.S.; Chaput, J.P.; Adamo, K.B.; Aubert, S.; Barnes, J.D.; Choquette, L.; Duggan, M.; Faulkner, G.; Goldfield, G.S.; Gray, C.E.; et al. Canadian 24-hour movement guidelines for the early years (0–4 years): An integration of physical activity, sedentary behaviour, and sleep. *BMC Public Health* **2017**, *17*, 874. [CrossRef] [PubMed]

39. Chaput, J.P.; Colley, R.C.; Aubert, S.; Carson, V.; Janssen, I.; Roberts, K.C.; Tremblay, M.S. Proportion of preschool-aged children meeting the Canadian 24-hour movement guidelines and associations with adiposity: Results from the Canadian health measures survey. *BMC Public Health* **2017**, *17*, 829. [CrossRef] [PubMed]

40. Roman-Vinas, B.; Chaput, J.P.; Katzmarzyk, P.T.; Fogelholm, M.; Lambert, E.V.; Maher, C.; Maia, J.; Olds, T.; Onywera, V.; Sarmiento, O.L.; et al. Proportion of children meeting recommendations for 24-hour movement guidelines and associations with adiposity in a 12-country study. *Int. J. Behav. Nutr. Phys. Act.* **2016**, *13*, 123. [CrossRef] [PubMed]

41. Li, Y.; Pan, A.; Wang, D.D.; Liu, X.; Dhana, K.; Franco, O.H.; Kaptoge, S.; Di Angelantonio, E.; Stampfer, M.; Willett, W.C.; et al. Impact of healthy lifestyle factors on life expectancies in the US population. *Circulation* **2018**. [CrossRef] [PubMed]

42. Kokkinos, P. Physical activity, health benefits, and mortality risk. *ISRN Cardiol.* **2012**, *2012*, 718789. [CrossRef] [PubMed]

43. Lee, I.M.; Skerrett, P.J. Physical activity and all-cause mortality: What is the dose-response relation? *Med. Sci. Sports Exerc.* **2001**, *33*, S459–S471. [CrossRef] [PubMed]

44. Stewart, R.A.H.; Held, C.; Hadziosmanovic, N.; Armstrong, P.W.; Cannon, C.P.; Granger, C.B.; Hagstrom, E.; Hochman, J.S.; Koenig, W.; Lonn, E.; et al. Physical activity and mortality in patients with stable coronary heart disease. *J. Am. Coll. Cardiol.* **2017**, *70*, 1689–1700. [CrossRef] [PubMed]

45. Leitzmann, M.F.; Park, Y.; Blair, A.; Ballard-Barbash, R.; Mouw, T.; Hollenbeck, A.R.; Schatzkin, A. Physical activity recommendations and decreased risk of mortality. *Arch. Intern. Med.* **2007**, *167*, 2453–2460. [CrossRef] [PubMed]

46. Barnekow-Bergkvist, M.; Hedberg, G.; Janlert, U.; Jansson, E. Prediction of physical fitness and physical activity level in adulthood by physical performance and physical activity in adolescence—An 18-year follow-up study. *Scand. J. Med. Sci. Sports* **1998**, *8*, 299–308. [CrossRef] [PubMed]

47. Twisk, J.W.; Van Mechelen, W.; Kemper, H.C.; Post, G.B. The relation between "long-term exposure" to lifestyle during youth and young adulthood and risk factors for cardiovascular disease at adult age. *J. Adolesc. Health* **1997**, *20*, 309–319. [CrossRef]

48. Corica, D.; Aversa, T.; Valenzise, M.; Messina, M.F.; Alibrandi, A.; De Luca, F.; Wasniewska, M. Does family history of obesity, cardiovascular, and metabolic diseases influence onset and severity of childhood obesity? *Front. Endocrinol.* **2018**, *9*, 187. [CrossRef] [PubMed]

49. Dobbs, R.; Sawers, C.; Thompson, F.; Manyika, J.; Woetzel, J.; Child, P.; McKenna, S.; Spatharou, A. *Overcoming Obesity: An Initial Economic Analysis*; McKinsey Global Institute, 2014.

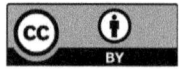

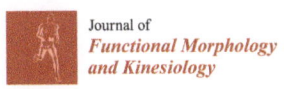
Journal of
Functional Morphology and Kinesiology

Editorial

Preventing Violence and Social Exclusion through Sport and Physical Activity: The SAVE Project

Ambra Gentile [1],*, Irena Valantine [2], Inga Staskeviciute-Butiene [2], Rasa Kreivyte [3], Dino Mujkic [4], Aela Ajdinovic [4], Ana Kezić [5], Đurđica Miletić [5], Almir Adi Kovačević [6], Dejan Madic [7], Patrik Drid [7] and Antonino Bianco [1]

[1] Department of Psychological, Pedagogical and Educational Sciences, University of Palermo, Viale delle Scienze, Ed. 15, 90128 Palermo, Italy; antonino.bianco@unipa.it

[2] Department of Sport Management, Economics and Sociology, Lithuanian Sports University; 44221 Kaunas, Lithuania; irena.valantine@lsu.lt (I.V.); inga.staskeviciute@lsu.lt (I.S.-B.)

[3] Department of Coaching Sciences, Lithuanian Sports University, Kaunas 44221, Lithuania; rasa.kreivyte@lsu.lt

[4] Faculty of Sport ad Physical Education, University of Sarajevo, Sarajevo 71000, Bosnia and Herzegovina; dmujkic@fasto.unsa.ba (D.M.); internationalfasto@gmail.com (A.A.)

[5] Faculty of Kinesiology, University of Split, 21000 Split, Croatia; anakezic@kifst.hr (A.K.); mileticd@kifst.hr (Đ.M.)

[6] World University Service (WUS) Austria, 8010 Graz, Austria; adi.kovacevic@wus-austria.org

[7] Faculty of Sport and Physical Education, University of Novi Sad, Novi Sad 21000, Serbia; dekimadic@gmail.com (D.M.); patrikdrid@gmail.com (P.D.)

* Correspondence: ambra.gentile91@gmail.com

Received: 28 March 2018; Accepted: 19 April 2018; Published: 21 April 2018

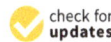
check for updates

Abstract: Sport Against Violence and Exclusion (SAVE), a project cofounded by the Erasmus + Program of the European Union, seeks to prevent violent and socially exclusive behaviors through physical activity. The current editorial shows a range of possible interpretations of these two phenomena from both a psychological and sociological point of view, offering helpful methods to coaches who train children (ages 6 to 12)in grass-root sport clubs. Following a thorough analysis, partners from seven EU countries (Lithuania, Italy, Croatia, Bosnia and Herzegovina, Serbia, Austria, and Spain) will be able to identify skills and techniques for coaches to ensure inclusive training methods as well as to provide them with effective conflict resolution tools. Furthermore, both trainers and parents will have access to an online platform with useful information regarding these issues.

Sport against Violence and Exclusion is a project cofounded by the Erasmus + Program of the European Union (Key action: Sport- 590711-EPP-1-2017-1-LT-SPO-SCP). The overall aim of the project is the prevention of violent and socially exclusive behaviors among youth in sport clubs. This goal can be achieved by enabling coaches from grass-root sport clubs to recognize these behaviors as well as the conflict resolution skills with which to address them. As stated by the Durban Declaration and Program of Action, sport and physical activity are promising instruments in the prevention of inequality, racism, and intolerance. Sport clubs are designed to be a valuable environment in which youth can learn respectful behaviors which are valid in every social context [1], and it is possible to define effective prevention strategies according to the psychological literature.

Concerning social exclusion, there is a positive relation between an individual's identification with a group and psychological wellness [2]: People who have been victims of social exclusion tend to suffer from negative emotions (sadness, disappointment, jealousy, anger, and shame) [3], depression [4], and tend to behave aggressively [5]. It is possible to contextualize social exclusion referring to social identity theory [6], in which a part of an individual's self-esteem is linked to their membership in a group. Identifying with a group allows individuals to make a distinction between the ingroup (group membership) and the outgroup (everyone who is not in their group).The exclusion of undesirable individuals helps to maintain a positive social identity [7]. Thus, a coach's task should be the promotion of a more inclusive and open environment.

According to social development theory [8], children learn how to give sense to the world by play. They adapt their behaviors in relation to the social norms that are valid in a specific social setting and develop a moral conscience through their interactions with significant adults. This can similarly be applicable on the sport field, in which they can internalize group expectations about respectful and disrespectful behaviors through interactions with their coach and teammates, shaping a sense of moral conscience. Accordingly, coaches should be able to guide children to achieve this result by learning specific practices which contribute to the development of a common system of values.

Furthermore, the prevention of violent behaviors may be achieved through the application of Hirschi's social bond theory [9]. The theory suggests that the promotion of an individual's social bonds leads to increased adherence to social norms, preventing violent or otherwise deviant behavior. Thus, coaches should focus on those practices which strengthen social bonds among team members.

Finally, according to social learning theory, children learn how to give sense to the world by observing and imitating adult behaviors [10]. From this perspective, coaches could provide positive behavioral patterns which children could observe and implement.

On the basis of these premises, the SAVE project will promote respect among youth from 6 to 12 years old in grass-root sport clubs, with the aim to prevent violent behavior and to enhance social inclusion and equal opportunities. The age range of 6–12, i.e., school age, was chosen as, during this period, children begin to spend considerable amounts of time with their peers as well as participate in sport clubs. The project will be developed over 30 months and will be implemented in seven European countries: Lithuania, Italy, Croatia, Bosnia and Herzegovina, Serbia, Austria, and Spain.

Since the project will involve individuals across numerous nations, each with its own cultural context of knowledge, social norms, and life habits, it will be necessary to conduct a desk analysis and at least seven focus groups per country. This will enable an ability to define which behaviors should be labeled as violent or socially exclusive. Each focus group will be conducted with 5 coaches of grass-root sports as well as 5 parents whose children participate in grass-root sports.

Next, in consultation with current psychological literature, the skills and competencies necessary for coaches will be defined. The results of this phase will be used to design a training phase with a specific curriculum and skill cards which coaches will implement.

Concurrent to the implementation phase, an online platform accessible to both coaches and parents will be designed to provide materials useful in addressing violent and socially exclusive behaviors. At the end of the implementation phase, the Training Kit will be finalized with the Sport against Violence and Exclusion Handbook as well as all the materials, findings, and statistics produced during the project.

The SAVE project confronts a relevant social issue. It can help to build a more aware society through the application of social norms which help to prevent violent and socially exclusive behaviors. In previous decades, few scientific studies provided a thorough understanding of these phenomena. Even now, additional practical strategies to prevent violent and socially exclusive behavior are needed from the scientific community. Thus, the SAVE project fits perfectly within this research scenario and, in our view, can significantly contribute in addressing this social need.

Conflicts of Interest: The authors declare no conflict of interest.

References

1. Mutz, M.; Baur, J. The Role of Sports for Violence Prevention: Sport Club Participation and Violent Behaviour among Adolescents. *Int. J. Sport Policy* **2009**, *1*, 305–321. [CrossRef]

2. Hutchison, P.; Abrams, D.; Christian, J. The Social Psychology of Exclusion. In *Multidisciplinary Handbook of Social Exclusion Research*; John Wiley & Sons: Hoboken, NJ, USA, 2007; p. 29.
3. Deci, E.L.; Ryan, R.M. A Motivational Approach to Self: Integration in Personality. *Nebr. Symp. Motiv.* **1991**, *38*, 237–288.
4. Vanderhorst, R.K.; McLaren, S. Social Relationships as Predictors of Depression and Suicidal Ideation in Older Adults. *Aging Ment. Health* **2005**, *9*, 517–525. [CrossRef] [PubMed]
5. Twenge, J.M.; Baumeister, R.F.; Tice, D.M.; Stucke, T.S. If You Can't Join Them, Beat Them: Effects of Social Exclusion on Aggressive Behavior. *J. Pers. Soc. Psychol.* **2001**, *81*, 1058. [CrossRef] [PubMed]
6. Tajfel, H.; Turner, C. The Social Identity Theory of Intergroup Behavior. In *Key Readings in Social Psychology. Political Psychology*; Jost, J.T., Sidanius, J., Eds.; Psychology Press: New York, NY, USA, 2004.
7. Yzerbyt, V.; Castano, E.; Leyens, J.-P.; Paladino, M.-P. The Primacy of the Ingroup: The Interplay of Entitativity and Identification. *Eur. Rev. Soc. Psychol.* **2000**, *11*, 257–295. [CrossRef]
8. Vygotskij, L.S. *Pensiero e Linguaggio. Ricerche Psicologiche*; Giunti: Firenze, Italy, 2007.
9. Hirschi, T. Social Bond Theory.In Criminological theory: Past to present. Roxbury: Los Angeles, CA, USA, 1998.
10. Bandura, A. Social-Learning Theory of Identificatory Processes. In *Handbook of Socialization Theory and Research*; Goslin, D.A., Ed.; Rand McNally & Company: Chicago, IL, USA, 1969; Volume 213, p. 262.

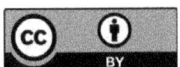

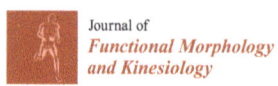

Journal of
Functional Morphology and Kinesiology

Editorial

Cognitive and Motivational Monitoring during Enriched Sport Activities in a Sample of Children Living in Europe. The Esa Program

Marianna Alesi [1,*], Carlos Silva [2], Carla Borrego [2], Diogo Monteiro [2], Rosario Genchi [3], Valentina Polizzi [3], Musa Kirkar [3], Yolanda Demetriou [4], Judith Brame [4], Fatma Neşe Şahin [5], Meltem Kızılyallı [5], Manuel Gómez-López [6], Guillermo López Sánchez [6], Simona Pajaujiene [7], Vinga Indriuniene [8], Ante Rađa [9] and Antonino Bianco [1]

1   Department of Psychological, Pedagogical and Educational Sciences, University of Palermo, Viale delle Scienze, Ed. 15, 90128 Palermo, Italy; antonino.bianco@unipa.it
2   Escola Superior de Desporto de Rio Maior (IPSantarém), Av. Dr. Mário Soares, 20413 RIO Maior, Portugal; csilva@esdrm.ipsantarem.pt (C.S.); ccborrego@esdrm.ipsantarem.pt (C.B.); diogomonteiro@esdrm.ipsantarem.pt (D.M.)
3   University of Palermo Sport Center (CUS Palermo), Via Altofonte, 80, 90129 Palermo, Italy; rosgenchi@gmail.com (R.G.); polizzivalentina26@gmail.com (V.P.); kirkar@ceipes.org (M.K.)
4   Department of School of Sport and Health Sciences, Technical University of Munich, Uptown Munich Campus D, Georg-Brauchle-Ring 60/62, 80992 Munich, Germany; yolanda.demetriou@tum.de (Y.D.); judith.brame@tum.de (J.B.)
5   Department of Sport and Health, Faculty of Sport Sciences, Ankara University, Golbaşı Yerleşkesi Spor Bilimleri Fakültesi, Golbaşı, 06830 Ankara, Turkey; nesehome@hotmail.com (F.N.S.); meltemkizilyalli@ankara.edu.tr (M.K.)
6   Department of Physical Activity and Sport, Faculty of Sports Sciences, University of Murcia, Calle Argentina, s/n., 30720 Murcia, Spain; mgomezlop@um.es (M.G.-L.); gfls@um.es (G.L.S.)
7   Department of Coaching Science, Lithuanian Sports University, Sporto 6, LT-44221 Kaunas, Lithuania; Simona.Pajaujiene@lsu.lt
8   Department of Health, Physical and Social Education Department, Lithuanian Sports University, Sporto 6, LT-44221 Kaunas, Lithuania vinga.indriuniene@lsu.lt
9   Faculty of Kinesiology, University of Split, Teslina 6, 21000 Split, Croatia; arada@kifst.hr
*   Correspondence: marianna.alesi@unipa.it; Tel.: +39-091-23899702

Received: 20 November 2017; Accepted: 8 December 2017; Published: 13 December 2017

Enriched Sport Activities (ESA) Program is an Evidence-based Practice Exercise Program cofounded by the Erasmus + Programme of the European Union (Key action: Sport-579661-EPP-1-2016-2-IT-SPO-SCP). It aims to enhance social inclusion, equal opportunities and psycho-physical wellbeing in children with typical development and special needs. This aim will be pursued through two ways: (1) Children and preadolescents' participation in Enriched Sport Activities (ESA) Program; (2) Parents' involvement and education on cognitive, motivational and social benefits of Physical Activities (PA) in their children.

Recent research showed that high-level cognitive processes, such as inhibition, shifting, working memory and planning, can be improved by aerobic exercise programs following both single bouts of exercise and longer trainings from moderate to vigorous intensity [1]. Nevertheless, in the developmental age, structured sport activities, such as martial arts, basketball, soccer, rowing and dancing, act by delivering both physical and psychological benefits. The former involve physical fitness such as cardiorespiratory fitness, muscular strength, muscular endurance, flexibility and motor skills such as coordination, whilst the latter concern enjoyment, self-confidence and self-esteem, a sense of belonging and social support [2–4]. The effectiveness of PMA (Programma Motorio Arricchito), a structured motor program on coordination and executive functioning in kindergarten children, has been demonstrated [5]. Moreover, exercise intervention trainings directed at increasing motor abilities in individuals with intellectual disabilities revealed to be efficacious to increase specific cognitive abilities such as reaction times [6,7].

Nevertheless, family stimulates children's participation in Physical Activity (PA) because of its key role to influence the choice of social and physical activities in childhood. Specifically, family influences the amount, the duration and the complexity of sport activities both in typically and atypically developing children by providing adequate scaffolding during collaborative performances as well as stimulating the sense of competence and the mastery motivation needed to cope challenging physical tasks [8,9].

On the basis of these theoretical premises, the ESA project aims at enhancing social inclusion, equal opportunities and psycho-physical wellbeing in children with typical development and special needs. It will be developed over three years and it involves a specialized practitioners team (coaches, sport scientists and psychologists) and the establishment of a European network among families, practitioners and schools. The intervention is carried out in seven European countries: Italy, Germany, Portugal, Spain, Lithuania, Croatia and Turkey.

According to the ESA Program aims, the TEG (Technical Expert Group) in charge with the Thematic Area 2 (TA2-cognitive functioning, sport motivation, social inclusion, equal opportunities and special needs) is focusing on a systematic literature review to provide the current evidence on the effects of PA programmes on enhancing children's and adolescents' motivation towards physical activity. Additionally, SOPs (Standard Operating Procedures) have been defined to select tests able to predict and monitor cognitive, social and motivational growth in a population target of children (6–14 years) living across Europe. The age range from 6–14 years was chosen because children's PA levels are acknowledged to decrease over this stage, with higher rates of drop-out in girls' population, but also because this is a critical phase to address precautionary intervention programs aimed at stimulating an active lifestyle able to prevent inactivity.

Starting from previous successful experiences, the TEG has implemented: (1) the Enriched Sport Activities (ESA) Program by adapting and enlarging previous successful experiences such as PMA and exercise intervention trainings [5]; (2) a Parent Education Program to train parents on cognitive, motivational and social benefits deriving from regular PA in childhood and establish educational models and strategies to improve participation in PA by their children. ESA is an integrated sport program in which 27 sessions of warm up in sport activities for typical children, such as soccer, track and field, swimming, basketball, handball and APA (Adapted Physical Activities) for children with special needs are enriched by cognitive tasks aimed at improving executive functions as working memory, shifting and inhibition processes. The Parent Education Program is composed of four sessions that will be carried out for each group of parents (10–12 max group members).

The aim is to provide, encourage and improve parents' strategies aimed at supporting motivation towards PA in their children. During "ESA Parent Education Program" the parents will be involved in group discussions about how to provide their children a climate characterized by high levels of support and patience, not to judge negative manifestations or the expression of negative affect concerning their children's sport performances, to encourage children to choose what they are more interested in and to choose what kind of sport activity is the best for their psycho-physic wellness.

Next step is the administration of the ESA Program and the Parent Education. To sum up, ESA Program aims at implementing guidelines to enhance cognitive abilities, motivation and participation in sport activities as natural and enjoyable instruments of growth. The final goal is to stimulate global development in children with typical development and special needs [10]. However, the main limitation of the program study is the future generalizability of the findings regarding the population with special needs because only two groups with special needs (children with Asthma and children with Down Syndrome) participate in the project. So, in the future the sample with special needs need to be enlarged.

Future contributions to the field are to establish a network approach involving educational agencies as families, practitioners and schools. This network approach has been chosen because traditional physical activity promotion interventions using individual approaches have revealed to be limited in long-term maintenance of benefits. After the project lifetime the web platform (ESA database, ESA cloud, ESA tasks, ESA smartphone apps, ESA school programs) will be available to be adopted for further European Union projects and initiative. In more details, every European citizen can easily visit the ESA Program web site and can discover the ESA aims, ESA research units, current researchers, reports, statistics and most important normative values and guidelines for best practices.

Conflicts of Interest: The authors declare no conflict of interest.

References

1. Davis, C.L.; Tomporowski, P.D.; McDowell, J.E.; Austin, B.P.; Miller, P.H.; Yanasak, N.E.; Allison, J.D.; Naglieri, J.A. Exercise Improves Executive Function and Achievement and Alters Brain Activation in Overweight Children: A Randomized Controlled Trial. *Health Psychol.* **2011**, *30*, 91–98. [CrossRef] [PubMed]
2. Haapala, E.A. Cardiorespiratory Fitness and Motor Skills in Relation to Cognition and Academic Performance in Children—A Review. *J. Hum. Kinet.* **2013**, *36*, 55–68. [CrossRef] [PubMed]
3. Diamond, A. Effects of Physical Exercise on Executive Functions: Going beyond Simply Moving to Moving with Thought. *Ann. Sports Med. Res.* **2015**, *2*, 1011. [PubMed]
4. Alesi, M.; Bianco, A.; Padulo, J.; Luppina, G.; Petrucci, M.; Paoli, A.; Palma, A.; Pepi, A. Motor and cognitive growth following a Football Training Program. *Front. Psychol.* **2015**, *6*, 162. [CrossRef] [PubMed]
5. Alesi, M.; Galassi, C.; Pepi, A. *Programma Motorio Arricchito. Educare allo Sviluppo Motorio e allo Sviluppo delle Funzioni Esecutive in età Prescolare*, 1th ed.; Edizioni Junior, Gruppo Spaggiari: Parma, Italy, 2016; ISBN 978-88-8434-778-7.
6. Alesi, M.; Battaglia, G.; Roccella, M.; Testa, D.; Palma, A.; Pepi, A. Improvement of gross motor and cognitive abilities by an exercise training program: Three case reports. *Neuropsychiatr. Dis. Treat.* **2014**, *10*, 479–485. [CrossRef] [PubMed]
7. Sundahl, L.; Zetterberg, M.; Wester, A.; Rehn, B.; Blomqvist, S. Physical Activity Levels among Adolescent and Young Adult Women and Men with and without Intellectual Disability. *J. Appl. Res. Intellect. Disabil.* **2016**, *29*, 93–98. [CrossRef] [PubMed]
8. Batey, C.A.; Missiuna, B.W.; Timmons, J.A.; Hay, B.E.; Faught, J.; Cairney, M. Self-efficacy toward physical activity and the physical activity behavior of children with and without Developmental Coordination Disorder. *Hum. Mov. Sci.* **2013**, *36*, 258–271. [CrossRef] [PubMed]
9. Alesi, M.; Pepi, A. Physical Activity Engagement in Young People with Down Syndrome: Investigating Parental Beliefs. *J. Appl. Res. Intellect. Disabil.* **2017**, *30*, 71–83. [CrossRef] [PubMed]
10. EU Commission: Special Eurobarometer 412. *Sport and Physical Activity*; Social, SEWETO, Ed.; EU Commission: Brussels, Belgium, 2014.

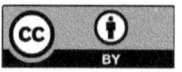

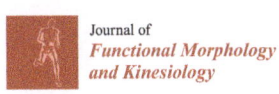

Journal of
*Functional Morphology
and Kinesiology*

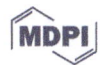

Article

Organized Sports and Physical Activities as Sole Influencers of Fitness: The Homeschool Population

Laura S. Kabiri *, Augusto X. Rodriguez, Amanda M. Perkins-Ball and Cassandra S. Diep

Kinesiology Department, Rice University, Houston, TX 77005, USA; augusto.x.rodriguez@rice.edu (A.X.R.); aperkinsball@rice.edu (A.M.P.-B.); csdiep@rice.edu (C.S.D.)
* Correspondence: laura.kabiri@rice.edu; Tel.: +1-713-718-2012

Received: 14 December 2018; Accepted: 25 January 2019; Published: 28 January 2019

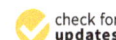

check for
updates

Abstract: Homeschool children may rely solely on organized sports and physical activities to achieve recommended levels of physical activity and fitness. The purpose of this study was to investigate differences in fitness levels between homeschool children who did, and did not, participate in organized sports or physical activities, and then examine relationships between hours per week in sports or physical activities and cardiorespiratory fitness as measured by portions of the FitnessGram® test battery. Organized sports/physical activity participation information was gathered on 100 children ages 10–17 years who completed tests of upper, abdominal, and cardiorespiratory fitness. The current investigation revealed that participation alone was not associated with higher levels of physical fitness as assessed by the 90° push-up test or curl-up test nor was time in participation related to cardiorespiratory fitness as assessed by the Progressive Aerobic Capacity Endurance Run (PACER). These activities alone may be insufficient for meeting physical activity recommendations and improving physical fitness. Therefore, children and adolescents educated at home may need additional opportunities to participate in unstructured daily physical activity.

Keywords: sport; conditioning; physical activity; children; adolescents

---

1. Introduction

Physical activity and fitness are critical for health and wellbeing. Specifically, participation in organized sports is a way for children and adolescents to get the recommended levels of physical activity [1] and has been recommended by the American Academy of Pediatrics as an opportunity for children and adolescents to increase their physical activity [2]. Defined as "an activity involving physical exertion and skill in which an individual or team competes against another or others for entertainment" [3], sports may include moderate (e.g., badminton, cricket) or vigorous-intensity physical activity (e.g., competitive swimming) [4]. Numerous studies have found sports participation to be beneficial for children and adolescent's psychological, social, and physical health [5–12].

A systematic review of the psychological and social benefits of participation in sports among youth revealed higher self-esteem, fewer depressive symptoms, higher confidence, and improved teamwork and social skills among sport participants than non-sport participants [5]. Sports participation was also related to beneficial health behaviors (e.g., fruit and vegetable consumption) [6], more positive attitudes and beliefs about physical activity [7], and physical activity levels [6]. These benefits may carry into adulthood, as sports participation in childhood and adolescence has been associated with physical activity levels in adulthood [13–16].

Cardiorespiratory and muscular fitness may also be improved with sports participation. In one study, U.S. adolescents who played school sports performed more pull-ups, had stronger grip strength, and performed the plank fitness test longer than those not in school sports [5]. School sports participation was also associated with improved performance on the 20-m shuttle run in a sample of Australian youth [8]. Outside of school, participation in sports outside school and participation in sports competitions were associated with better performances on the 20-m shuttle run in a sample of youth in Portugal [9,10]. Children from Denmark, who participated in gymnastics, handball, tennis, and swimming, had high levels of anaerobic power and muscular strength [11]. Another study of ninth-grade girls in the U.S. specifically found that, those who participated on at least two sports teams (either in school or outside school), performed better on the step test than those who did not participate in any sports [12]. Further, adolescent females in cycling, running, and swimming [17] and adolescent males in various high-impact sports (e.g., football, rugby, and hockey) [18] had higher bone mineral density.

Despite existing research on the benefits of participation in organized sports among children and adolescents, one population that has been overlooked in such research is homeschool children and adolescents, who may be at increased risk for cardiovascular disease and adiposity [19]. Unlike public school children, homeschool children do not regularly participate in school-based physical activity (e.g., physical education, recess, school sports) because they are not subject to state regulations for physical education classes, physical activity initiatives, or fitness testing [19]. Thus, organized sports and organized physical activities may be the only avenues through which homeschool children engage in purposeful exercise.

With an increasing prevalence of homeschooling and home education around the world (including almost 2 million children in the U.S. [19]), and the lack of regulations for physical education, research is needed to investigate whether organized sports and physical activities alone are sufficient to improve fitness in homeschool youth. Thus, the purpose of this study was to investigate differences in fitness levels between homeschool children who did and did not participate in organized sports or physical activities. A secondary purpose was to examine any relationships between average hours per week in sports or physical activities and cardiorespiratory fitness. Given previous research on the relationship between sports and fitness, we hypothesized that homeschool children who participated in organized sports or physical activities would have improved fitness over those who did not participate in organized sports or physical activities, and that more hours would be related to improved cardiorespiratory fitness.

2. Materials and Methods

Participant recruitment and data collection occurred after ethical approval from the Institutional Review Board (Protocol #18919 and #19736) of Texas Woman's University on 3 March 2016 and 19 January 2017 respectively as part of Fitness Assessment in the Homeschool: The F.A.I.T.H. Study—Part I and II. Homeschool children ages 5–17 years were recruited from the Greater Houston area through email, homeschool groups, and word of mouth. A subset of this population (ages 10–17 years) was intended for use in this study due to lack of normative data for younger children on selected outcome measures. An *a priori* power analysis with an alpha of 0.05, power of 0.8, and effect size of 0.3 revealed a necessary sample size of 88 participants.

Parents completed a survey including information on whether their child was currently participating in organized sports or physical activities (yes/no). If the answer was yes, the parent was asked to provide the average number of hours of participation per week. For the purposes of this study, organized participation was defined as any sport or physical activity in which the child paid to participate.

To assess multiple aspects of physical fitness, all participants completed the 90° push-up test, curl-up test, and Progressive Aerobic Capacity Endurance Run (PACER) as part of the FitnessGram® test battery (v. 10.0; Human Kinetics, Champaign, IL, USA). The 90° push-up test is a measure of upper body strength and endurance while the curl-up test assesses abdominal strength and endurance. The PACER is a test of cardiorespiratory fitness and is administered similar to the 20-m shuttle run or 20-m beep test [20]. The FitnessGram® test battery has been shown to be both reliable and valid in this population and is routinely employed in American public schools [21–23]. All tests were administered as per the FitnessGram® administration manual and performed until two failed repetitions or volitional exhaustion, whichever occurred first [20].

Results for each test portion (90° push-up, curl-up, PACER) were dichotomized into healthy or needs improvement classifications. The PACER was also used to calculate an age and gender specific estimated VO_{2max} for each participant to measure cardiorespiratory fitness in addition to the dichotomized classification. All results and classifications were calculated using age and gender specific normative data provided by FitnessGram®. This was done to account for the effects of both age and gender on test results.

Chi-square tests were used to explore statistically significant differences in fitness between children who did and did not participate in organized sports or physical activities. Comparisons were made between participation groups for overall fitness (healthy rating for all three tests) as well as for a healthy classification on each individual test (90° push-up, curl-up, PACER). Pearson correlation coefficient was used to determine any relationship between average hours per week of organized sports or physical activity and cardiorespiratory fitness (VO_{2max}). All statistical analyses were done using IBM SPSS Statistics for Windows (v. 25.0; IBM, Corporation, Armonk, NY, USA) with an alpha level of $p = 0.05$ used to indicate statistical significance.

3. Results

3.1. Participant Demographics

A total of 211 participants aged 5–17 years enrolled in the study. Of those, 100 participants met the age requirement (10–17 years) for this portion of the study. This subset ($n = 100$) of age-appropriate participants was used for all data analyses. Participant characteristics can be found in Table 1; Table 2. The sample was evenly split between genders with an average age of 12.71 years. They were predominantly non-Hispanic white and of normal body mass index.

Table 1. Frequencies for participant characteristics.

Variable	n	Percent
Gender		
Male	50	50%
Female	50	50%
Total	100	100%
Ethnicity		
Non-Hispanic White	83	83%
Hispanic	5	5%
Non-Hispanic Black	5	5%
Asian	3	3%
Other	4	4%
Total	100	100%

Note: n: 100.

Table 2. Descriptive characteristics for physiological characteristics.

Variable	n	Mean	SD
Age (years)	100	12.71	2.17
Years in homeschool	100	5.80	2.85
Hours per week in sports participation	100	4.68	3.60
Curl-up repetitions	100	15.82	15.80
Push-up repetitions	100	16.47	8.078
PACER laps	100	35.16	18.08
Estimated VO_{2max}	100	43.78	6.23

Table 2. *Cont.*

BMI Classification	*n*	Percent
Under weight	3	3%
Normal weight	81	81%
Overweight	10	10%
Obese	6	6%
Total	100	100%

Note: *n*: 100.

3.2. Outcomes

Overall, 80% of participants (*n* = 80) were currently engaged in some form of organized sports participation or physical activity. Healthy classification overall and for each individual test can be seen in Table 3 while specific test performance details are in Table 2. The sample had a mean of 4.68 h/week of sports participation (Range = 0–17; SD = 3.60) with a majority exhibiting good upper body strength and endurance as well as cardiorespiratory fitness.

Table 3. Sports participation and healthy status frequencies.

Sports Participation	*n*	Percent
Yes	80	80%
No	20	20%
Total	100	100%
Overall Healthy Classification		
Unhealthy in at least one	77	77%
Healthy in all three	23	23%
Total	100	100%
Curl-up Healthy Classification		
Needs improvement	63	63%
Healthy	37	37%
Total	100	100%
Push-up Healthy Classification		
Needs improvement	15	15%
Healthy	85	85%
Total	100	100%
PACER Healthy Classification		
Needs improvement	33	33%
Healthy	67	67%
Total	100	100%

Note: *n*: 100.

Chi-square tests revealed no significant (χ^2 (1, *n* = 100) = 0.903 *p* = 0.342.) difference between participation groups for overall fitness as seen in Table 4. These results indicate no association between participating in organized sports or physical activity and being in the healthy fitness zone in all three categories. Additional chi-square tests found similar non-significant differences between groups for a healthy classification on each individual test as well (90° push-up: χ^2 (1, *n* = 100) = 0.490, *p* = 0.484; curl-up: χ^2 (1, *n* = 100) = 0.526, *p* = 0.468; PACER: χ^2 (1, *n* = 100) = 0.005, *p* = 0.942). Pearson correlation revealed a non-significant relationship between average hours per week of organized sports or physical activity and estimated VO_{2max} (*r* = 0.121, *p* = 0.230).

Table 4. Crosstab analysis.

Variable	No	Yes	Total
Unhealthy in one	17	60	77
Healthy in all	3	20	23
Total	20	80	100

	Value	df	Sig.
Pearson Chi-Square	0.903	1	0.342

Notes: df (degree of freedom): 1; Sig.: $p = 0.05$.

4. Discussion

The primary findings of this study demonstrated no relationship between participation in organized sports and physical fitness among homeschool children and adolescents. The majority of subjects participated in some form of organized sport or physical activity. However, participants did not have higher levels of overall fitness (i.e., achieved a healthy rating for all three tests) or for each individual test (i.e., 90° push-up, curl-up, PACER) than non-participants. Furthermore, there was no relationship between number of hours spent participating in sport each week and cardiorespiratory fitness. These findings were in direct opposition to our original hypotheses.

Previous studies have provided evidence supporting the relationship between sport participation and physical fitness indicators among children and adolescents [8]. High levels of cardiorespiratory endurance, muscular strength and endurance, and power among girls and boys participating in a variety of sports, including tennis, gymnastics, handball, and swimming, have been well documented [10,11]. Further, studies examining running and high-volume loading sports, such as soccer, basketball, tennis, and rugby, have been associated with higher bone mineral density [17,18].

While previous research has found positive associations between sport and fitness, the results of our study suggest sport participation alone may not be enough to achieve desired levels health-related physical fitness. This may be because the achievement of physical activity recommendations is important for developing physical fitness [24]. The World Health Organization (WHO) suggests children and youth ages 5–17 accumulate a minimum of 60 min of primarily aerobic moderate—to vigorous-intensity physical activity (MVPA) daily, as well as muscle- and bone-strengthening activities at least three days per week, in order to improve health and physical fitness [25].

Participation in organized sport alone may be insufficient for children in order for them to meet daily physical activity guidelines for several reasons, including not participating in MVPA outside of sport practices, not practicing frequently, or practices being low in MVPA [26]. Recent analyses of youth sport practices revealed that children engaged in MVPA 34–50% of their time spent in practice [26–29], which is approximately 20–30 min (one-third to one-half) of MVPA toward daily public health guidelines [26,27]. When exploring varied practice structures and time segments in youth flag football, Schleter and colleagues [27] found that free-play, game-play, and warmup segments resulted in greater percentages of time spent in MVPA than scrimmage, strategy, and sport-skill segments of practice. A number of contextual variables may contribute to low amounts of MVPA during a practice session, such as those related to tasks (e.g., time devoted to organizational tasks, strategy, or self-care), and setting (e.g., fewer opportunities to participate in relation to children available to participate) [27]. Recent interventions have implemented strategies in effort to address these factors to increase MVPA during youth sport practices [29,30].

To the best of our knowledge, no previous studies have examined the relationship between sports participation and achievement of health-related physical fitness among homeschool children and adolescents. Strengths of the study include a sample size exceeding the required number of participants determined by an a priori power analysis, as well as the broad age range and even gender representation of our population. Recruitment of children not currently participating in physical education classes through the public-school system also strengthens our findings by focusing solely on effects of organized sports and activities. Limitations of the study include assessment of organized sports and physical activity participation by parental report only and failure to further qualify or classify the type of participation. In addition, participants consisted of majority healthy weight children and adolescents; therefore, the sample did not allow the researchers to control for obesity, a known confounding variable. Further, the study did not quantify participants' habitual physical activity. Previous studies investigating the effects of habitual physical activity on fitness among children and adolescents have yielded mixed results [31]. Future studies should attempt to more accurately quantify the amount of sport practice time spent engaged in MVPA.

5. Conclusions

The current investigation revealed that organized sport participation and/or physical activity alone was not associated with higher levels of physical fitness among 10–17 year old homeschool students. These activities alone may be insufficient for meeting MVPA recommendations and improving physical fitness. Therefore, children and adolescents educated at home may need additional opportunities to participate in unstructured physical activity daily.

Author Contributions: Individual author contributions are as follows: conceptualization, L.S.K., C.S.D., A.M.P.-B. and A.X.R.; investigation, L.S.K.; project administration, L.S.K.; methodology, L.S.K.; formal analysis, A.X.R.; writing—original draft preparation, L.S.K., C.S.D., A.M.P.-B., and A.X.R.; writing—review and editing, L.S.K., C.S.D., A.M.P.-B., and A.X.R.; funding acquisition, L.S.K.

Funding: This research was funded in part by the Texas Physical Therapy Foundation.

Acknowledgments: A portion of this research was conducted by Laura S. Kabiri at Texas Woman's University in her role as a graduate student. We would like to acknowledge Wayne Brewer, Alexis Ortiz, and Katy Mitchell (chair) for their role on the dissertation committee.

Conflicts of Interest: The authors declare no conflict of interest. The funders had no role in the design of the study; in the collection, analyses, or interpretation of data; in the writing of the manuscript, or in the decision to publish the results.

References

1. Micheli, L.; Mountjoy, M.; Engebretsen, L.; Hardman, K.; Kahlmeier, S.; Lambert, E.; Ljungqvist, A.; Matsudo, V.; McKay, H.; Sundberg, C.J. Fitness and health of children through sport: The context for action. *Br. J. Sports Med.* **2011**, *45*, 931–936. [CrossRef] [PubMed]
2. Washington, R.L.; Bernhardt, D.T.; Gomez, J.; Johnson, M.D.; Martin, T.J.; Rowland, T.W.; Small, E.; LeBlanc, C.; Krein, C.; Malina, R.; et al. Organized sports for children and preadolescents. *Pediatrics* **2001**, *107*, 1459–1462. [PubMed]
3. Sport. Available online: https://en.oxforddictionaries.com/definition/sport (accessed on 12 December 2018).
4. Somerset, S.; Hoare, D.J. Barriers to voluntary participation in sport for children: A systematic review. *BMC Pediatr.* **2018**, *18*, 47. [CrossRef] [PubMed]
5. Eime, R.M.; Young, J.A.; Harvey, J.T.; Charity, M.J.; Payne, W.R. A systematic review of the psychological and social benefits of participation in sport for children and adolescents: Informing development of a conceptual model of health through sport. *Int. J. Behav. Nutr. Phys. Act.* **2013**, *10*, 98. [CrossRef]
6. Pate, R.R.; Trost, S.G.; Levin, S.; Dowda, M. Sports participation and health-related behaviors among US youth. *Arch. Pediatr. Adolesc. Med.* **2000**, *154*, 904–911. [CrossRef]
7. Loprinzi, P.D.; Cardinal, B.J.; Cardinal, M.K.; Corbin, C.B. Physical education and sport: Does participation relate to physical activity patterns, observed fitness, and personal attitudes and beliefs? *Am. J. Health Promot.* **2018**, *32*, 613–620. [CrossRef]
8. Telford, R.M.; Telford, R.D.; Cochrane, T.; Cunningham, R.B.; Olive, L.S.; Davey, R. The influence of sport club participation on physical activity, fitness and body fat during childhood and adolescence: The LOOK longitudinal study. *J. Sci. Med. Sport* **2016**, *19*, 400–406. [CrossRef]

9.   Aires, L.; Silva, G.; Martins, C.; Santos, M.P.; Ribeiro, J.C.; Mota, J. Influence of activity patterns in fitness during youth. *Int. J. Sports Med.* **2012**, *33*, 325–329. [CrossRef]
10. Silva, G.; Andersen, L.B.; Aires, L.; Mota, J.; Oliveira, J.; Ribeiro, J.C. Associations between sports participation, levels of moderate to vigorous physical activity and cardiorespiratory fitness in children and adolescents. *J. Sports Sci.* **2013**, *31*, 1359–1367. [CrossRef]
11. Bencke, J.; Damsgaard, R.; Saekmose, A.; Jørgensen, P.; Jørgensen, K.; Klausen, K. Anaerobic power and muscle strength characteristics of 11 years old elite and non-elite boys and girls from gymnastics, team handball, tennis and swimming. *Scand. J. Med. Sci. Sports* **2002**, *12*, 171–178. [CrossRef]
12. Phillips, J.A.; Young, D.R. Past-year sports participation, current physical activity, and fitness in urban adolescent girls. *J. Phys. Act. Health* **2009**, *6*, 105–111. [CrossRef] [PubMed]
13. Tammelin, T.; Näyhä, S.; Hills, A.P.; Järvelin, M.R. Adolescent participation in sports and adult physical activity. *Am. J. Prev. Med.* **2003**, *24*, 22–28. [CrossRef]
14. Aarnio, M.; Winter, T.; Peltonen, J.; Kujala, U.M.; Kaprio, J. Stability of leisure-time physical activity during adolescence—A longitudinal study among 16-, 17- and 18-year-old Finnish youth. *Scand. J. Med. Sci. Sports* **2002**, *12*, 179–185. [CrossRef] [PubMed]
15. Kjønniksen, L.; Anderssen, N.; Wold, B. Organized youth sport as a predictor of physical activity in adulthood. *Scand. J. Med. Sci. Sports* **2009**, *5*, 646–654. [CrossRef] [PubMed]
16. Telama, R.; Yang, X.; Hirvensalo, M.; Raitakari, O. Participation in organized youth sport as a predictor of adult physical activity: A 21-Year longitudinal study. *Pediatr. Exerc. Sci.* **2006**, *18*, 76–88. [CrossRef]
17. Duncan, C.S.; Blimkie, C.J.; Cowell, C.T.; Burke, S.T.; Briody, J.N.; Howman-Giles, R. Bone mineral density in adolescent female athletes: Relationship to exercise type and muscle strength. *Med. Sci. Sports Exerc.* **2002**, *34*, 286–294. [CrossRef]
18. Ginty, F.; Rennie, K.L.; Mills, L.; Steer, S.; Jones, S.; Prentice, A. Positive, site-specific associations between bone mineral status, fitness, and time spent at high-impact activities in 16- to 18-year-old boys. *Bone* **2005**, *36*, 101–110. [CrossRef]
19. Kabiri, L.S.; Mitchell, K.; Brewer, W.; Ortiz, A. How healthy is homeschool? An analysis of body composition and cardiovascular disease risk. *J. Sch. Health* **2018**, *88*, 132–138. [CrossRef]
20. Meredith, M.D.; Welk, G.J. *Fitnessgram and Activitygram Test Administration Manual*, 4th ed.; Human Kinetics: Champaign, IL, USA, 2013; ISBN 0-7360-9992-1.
21. Plowman, S.A.; Meredith, M.D. *Fitnessgram and Activitygram Reference Guide*, 4th ed.; The Cooper Institute: Dallas, TX, USA, 2013.
22. Mahar, M.; Rowe, D. Practical guidelines for valid and reliable youth fitness testing. *Meas. Phys. Educ. Exerc. Sci.* **2008**, *12*, 126–145. [CrossRef]
23. Artero, E.G.; España-Romero, V.; Castro-Piñero, J.; Ortega, F.B.; Suni, J.; Castilla-Garzon, M.J.; Ruiz, J.R. Reliability of field-based fitness tests in youth. *Int. J. Sports Med.* **2011**, *32*, 159–169. [CrossRef]
24. Morrow, J.R.; Tucker, J.S.; Jackson, A.W.; Martin, S.B.; Greenleaf, C.A.; Petrie, T.A. Meeting physical activity guidelines and health-related fitness in youth. *Am. J. Prev. Med.* **2013**, *44*, 439–444. [CrossRef] [PubMed]
25. WHO Physical Activity and Young People. Available online: https://www.who.int/dietphysicalactivity/factsheet_young_people/en/ (accessed on 11 December 2018).
26. Ridley, K.; Zabeen, S.; Lunnay, B.K. Children's physical activity levels during organised sports practices. *J. Sci. Med. Sport* **2018**, *21*, 930–934. [CrossRef] [PubMed]
27. Schlechter, C.R.; Guagliano, J.M.; Rosenkranz, R.R.; Milliken, G.A.; Dzewaltowski, D.A. Physical activity patterns across time-segmented youth sport flag football practice. *BMC Public. Health* **2018**, *18*. [CrossRef] [PubMed]
28. Leek, D.; Carlson, J.A.; Cain, K.L.; Henrichon, S.; Rosenberg, D.; Patrick, K.; Sallis, J.F. Physical activity during youth sports practices. *Arch. Pediatr. Adolesc. Med.* **2011**, *165*, 294–299. [CrossRef] [PubMed]
29. Guagliano, J.M.; Richard, R.R.; Kolt, G.S. Girls' physical activity levels during organized sports in Australia. *Med. Sci. Sports Exerc.* **2013**, *45*, 116–122. [CrossRef] [PubMed]

30. Guagliano, J.M.; Lonsdale, C.; Kolt, G.S.; Rosenkranz, R.R.; George, E.S. Increasing girls' physical activity during a short-term organized youth sport basketball program: A randomized controlled trial. *J. Sci. Med. Sport* **2015**, *18*, 412–417. [CrossRef] [PubMed]
31. Armstrong, N.; Tomkinson, G.R.; Ekelund, U. Aerobic fitness and its relationship to sport, exercise training and habitual physical activity during youth. *Br. J. Sports Med.* **2011**, *45*, 849–858. [CrossRef] [PubMed]

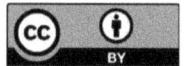

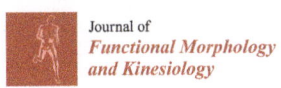

Journal of
Functional Morphology and Kinesiology

Article

School-Based Intervention on Cardiorespiratory Fitness in Brazilian Students: A Nonrandomized Controlled Trial

Giseli Minatto [1,*], Edio Luiz Petroski [2], Kelly Samara da Silva [1] and Michael J. Duncan [3]

1   Research Centre in Physical Activity and Health, School of Sports, Department of Physical Education Federal University of Santa Catarina, Campus Universitário—Trindade, Florianópolis, SC 88040-900, Brazil; kelly.samara@ufsc.br
2   Research Centre for Kineantropometry and Human Performan, School of Sports, Department of Physical Education Federal University of Santa Catarina, Campus Universitário—Trindade, Florianópolis, SC 88040-900, Brazil; edioluizpetroski@gmail.com
3   School of Life Sciences, Faculty of Health and Life Sciences, Coventry University, James Starley Building, Priory Street, Coventry, CV1 5FB, UK; aa8396@coventry.ac.uk
*   Correspondence: gminatto@gmail.com; Tel.: +55-48-3721-6342

Received: 19 December 2018; Accepted: 17 January 2019; Published: 21 January 2019

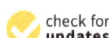

check for updates

Abstract: Background: In response to the worldwide increasing prevalence of low cardiorespiratory fitness (CRF), several interventions have been developed. The aim of this study was to examine the effect of a school-based intervention on CRF in Brazilian students. Methods: A nonrandomised controlled design tested 432 students (intervention group: $n = 247$) from 6th to 9th grade recruited from two public secondary schools in Florianopolis, in 2015. The intervention entitled *"MEXA-SE"* (move yourself), applied over 13 weeks, included four components: (1) increases in physical activity during Physical Education classes; (2) active recess; (3) educational sessions; and (4) educational materials. CRF (20-m shuttle run test) was the primary outcome. Results: The effect size of the intervention on CRF was 0.15 (CI 95% = –0.04; 0.34). In the within-group comparisons, VO2max decreased significantly from baseline to follow-up in the control group but remained constant in the intervention group. After adjustment variables, differences between intervention and control group were not statistically significant ($p > 0.05$). Conclusion: The *"MEXA-SE"* intervention did not have an effect on adolescents' CRF. However, maintenance of VO2max in intervention group and a reduction within control group demonstrates that this intervention may be beneficial for long-term CRF and, possibly, the increased intervention time could result in a better effect.

Keywords: physical fitness; children; adolescents; intervention study; physical education; school health; motor activity

---

1. Introduction

Cardiorespiratory fitness (CRF) is considered an important marker of health in childhood and adolescence [1]. Low CRF has been associated with increased cardiovascular disease risk in young people [2] and adults [3]. Similarly, the maintenance of adequate CRF has been considered a protective factor for reducing the burden of mortality from cardiovascular diseases [4].

In response to the worldwide increasing prevalence of low CRF, several interventions have been developed and evaluated in recent decades [5,6]. However, the evidence of the effectiveness of school-based interventions for the promotion of CRF in low-and middle-income countries (LMICs) is limited [6,7]. Interventions implemented in the school environment prioritising CRF suggest that, regardless of study design and of the test used to measure CRF, the largest effects on CRF were found as a result of greater session length (>60 min), frequency of three weekly sessions, programmes lasting from 13 to 24 weeks [6], and higher-intensity physical activity (PA) [5]. The literature also points to high-intensity interval training (HIIT) as a feasible and time-efficient approach for improving CRF in adolescent populations [8]. However, the embedding of HIIT within the school day (e.g., in physical education or activities adapted for the classroom) is limited [8].

In terms of intervention strategies administered within the school day, systematic reviews suggest that engagement in PA is one of the major strategies to improve CRF, with the school being a favourable environment for this [5,6]. The methods used to improve CRF via PA include increasing the number and intensity of physical education (PE) lessons a week; inclusion of aerobic and resistance exercises; increasing PA within and outside school [6]; and a combination of printed educational materials and changes to the school curriculum [5]. Interventions which include changes to both PE classes and another aspect of school provision (e.g., strategies of exercise/PA (effect size = 0.88; CI 95% 0.55; 1.24), PA after school time (effect size = 0.44; CI 95% 0.00; 0.87)) have reported a greater effect compared to solely PE-based strategies (effect size = 0.14; CI 95% −0.03; 0.31) [6]. In this context, we applied an intervention based on the evidence previously cited, adapted to the context of schools in Southern Brazil, a low- and middle-income country (LMIC). Thus, the present study aimed to examine the effect of a school-based intervention on CRF among Brazilian students.

2. Materials and Methods

2.1. Design and Participants

The "MEXA-SE" intervention was a nonrandomised controlled trial conducted in two (one experimental) secondary major schools of the South region of Brazil. Umbrella research had the objective of analysing the effect of a multicomponent intervention, applied during one school semester (approximately four months), on health-related physical fitness and body image of students from 6th to 9th grade. A detailed description of the full trial protocol can be accessed in the trial registration (Available online: https://www.clinicaltrials.gov/ct2/show/NCT02719704?term=NCT02719704&rank=1).

According to the records of the Municipal Department of Education in 2015, 7484 students from 6th to 9th grade were enrolled in 26 public schools. The sample size calculation considered the following parameters: Effect size (ES) for each outcome, power of 80%, and significance level of 5% (Table S1). Specifically, the calculation of the sample size for CRF required 35 people within each group, with an effect size of 0.68 [6]. To account for a potential 30% loss at follow-up, 46 participants per school were necessary. Following these parameters, the sample was calculated for all primary outcomes of the umbrella research. The largest sample size required among all outcomes was 295 students (see Table S1), and this was the minimum sample established for the recruitment of schools.

School recruitment was based on the identification of the larger sample size (n = 295) and on the agreement of PE teachers in the intervention school to participate in the intervention. Of the 26 existing schools identified, five were eligible, two located in the Southern region (about 689 students) and three in the North (about 1165 students). For this study, the two schools (one control and one experimental) were selected in the same region of the city (Northern region) in order to reduce the possible socioeconomic disparities among students (mean of total monthly income of the people responsible for the house of each census tract of schools in Northern region = R$273,321 (approximately $73,473; €64,160) and Southern region = R$707,416) (approximately $190,166; €166,060)) [9]. Of the selected schools, one refused to participate and the third school from the same region was invited to participate. Contact with these schools was initiated in December 2014. The allocation of schools in the intervention (IG) and control (CG) groups was determined by authorities of the Municipal Secretariat of Education and the researchers had no influence in this decision. All participating schools were located within the urban perimeter of Florianopolis and most of the students resided near the school.

All students from grade 6th to 9th of these schools were eligible (n = 1,011) (records of the Municipal Department of Education). The final sample size adopted was 295 students (see Table S1);

however, for ethical reasons and at the request of the principals of each school, the intervention was conducted with all students in the schools. In the intervention school, all students could participate in the activities offered in the *"MEXA-SE"* (move yourself) programme. In both the intervention and the control school, only the students who delivered parental permission were evaluated.

2.2. Intervention

2.2.1. Theoretical Aspects

The intervention strategies were developed considering previous evidence obtained via systematic review with meta-analysis [6] prepared for this purpose. The meta-analysis variables considered were CRF (primary outcome); intervention setting (school only); and strategies in intervention (actions in PE classes and one other) and control (traditional PE classes) groups. Additionally, the type of exercise for the IG (aerobic and resistance) was considered, along with session duration (minimum 45 min), weekly frequency (three times), and duration of intervention (13 weeks or more).

Intervention strategies (Table 1) related to PA were developed according to the theories of health promoting schools [10], sociocognitive theory [11], and the ecological model of health promotion [12]. Body image intervention was based on the sociocognitive theory [11] and the health belief model [13], and nutritional intervention was based on the dialogical model of health education [14]. The logical model of intervention (Figure S1) was developed in accordance with the suggestions of the Center for Disease Control and Prevention [15]. The logic model includes inputs available, developed activities, outputs, influencing factors, outcomes expected in the short and long term, and the desired aim of the intervention.

Table 1. Description of *"MEXA-SE"* actions.

Actions	Influence Level	Theory	No. Sessions	Duration	WF	Executing Agent
Training for PE teachers	School	EPS	1	4 h	-	Researchers (PE)
PE Classes: Stretching exercises (10 min), strength and muscular resistance (10 min), and increased intensity in the main part of the class (MVPA)	Individual	Meta-analysis	42 *	45 min	3	School PE teachers
Active recess	Individual, School	EPS; TSC; Meta-analysis	70 *	15 min	5	Researchers and School
Educational sessions on the following topics: Health, lifestyle, physical activity, and sedentary behaviour	Individual	EPS; TSC	2	45 min	†	School PE teachers
Educational sessions on healthy eating and nutrition	Individual	MDES	6	100 min	1	Researchers (Nutritionist)
Educational sessions related to body image	Individual	TSC; Belief in health	4	45 min	1	Researchers (PE)
Placement of posters about physical activity and sedentary behaviour in school and health units	School	EPS; MSE	-	-	†	Researchers, students and teachers
Distribution of leaflets on physical activity and sedentary behaviour	Individual, Family	EPS; MSE	-	-	††	School PE teachers Researchers

PE: Physical education; WF: Weekly frequency; MVPA: Moderate to vigorous physical activity; EPS: Health-Promoting Schools [10]; Meta-analysis [6]; TSC: Sociocognitive theory [11]; MSE: Ecological social model [12]; MDES: Dialogical model of health education [14]; * We considered 14 weeks of intervention; † fixed in the 3rd and 5th week of the intervention; †† delivered to students on the 3rd and 5th week of intervention and to parents on the 4th and 6th week.

2.2.2. Intervention Strategies

The intervention employed in the current study had four integrated components that were delivered during school time in a PE class or other module.

First Component: PE Classes

The first component was to increase time spent on in moderate to vigorous PA (MVPA) during the three PE lessons per week. The three weekly classes were conducted by PE teachers in the school. The lessons were composed of approximately 10 min of stretching exercises, 10 min of strength exercises/muscular endurance, and 20 min of aerobic exercise, prioritising activities that arouse students' interest and in which most of them were involved in movement. The content was organised according to the Curriculum Proposal for PE of Florianopolis [16] and the National Curriculum Parameters of PE [17]. Thus, we used different content from PE (games, sports, dancing, martial arts, gymnastics) and prioritised playful aspects of learning. In total, students received an average of 25 (SD = 6.4) PE lessons (45 min per lesson).

Second Component: Active Recess

Students were also encouraged to increase PA practice during school recess. Volleyball, basketball, football, futsal, handball, and ropes were available for students to occupy the school recess time actively. These materials could be used on the school environment, such as sports courts.

Third Component: Educational Sessions

Educational sessions on "Health, Lifestyle, Physical Activity and Sedentary Behaviour": These sessions were planned by researchers and conducted by school PE teachers and lasted 45 min each. The first session aimed to discuss issues related to health and healthy lifestyle, seeking to identify beneficial and harmful health behaviours. The second session was aimed at discussing PA, physical exercise, and sedentary behaviour, seeking to identify the physical activities practised by students, clarifying concepts, demonstrating the importance of each behaviour for health, and reflecting on changes that everyone could do to become more active. For the development of sessions, video, educational games, and posters were used.

Educational sessions on nutrition: These sessions consisted of six sessions (45 min per session) designed to promote reflection and positive changes in eating habits and healthcare (to improve knowledge and eating habits), conducted by a nutritionist with each school year group separately. The topics developed in the sessions were: (1) Healthy eating; (2) general recommendations about the choice of foods in terms of natural and processed meals; (3) consuming a wide variety of organically grown fruit and vegetables; (4) guidelines on how to combine foods in a meal; (5) guidelines on the act of eating; and (6) a cookery workshop. The teaching methods used were movies, expository lectures, workshop context posters, music, and cooking workshops.

Educational sessions on body image: These sessions comprised three sessions (45 min per session) focused on body image satisfaction conducted by a PE researcher. The topics developed in the sessions were: (1) Beauty standards; (2) individual qualities; and (3) preparation of a poster on the theme: "What is beauty to you?". The teaching methods used were movies, expository lectures, and workshop context posters. The intervention was delivered to each class (*n* = 18) separately.

Fourth Component: Education Materials

Leaflets about sedentary behaviour and PA outcomes were distributed at the school, and two folders were sent to the parents (Figure S2) by students. The first folder had messages about reducing sedentary behaviour (recommendations, tips for changing of this behaviour, etc.), and the second on increasing PA (the importance of parental incentive, examples and benefits of active living for youths).

The folders were also given by the PE teacher to the students with messages specific (Figure S3), along with educational sessions on these behaviours (third and fifth weeks).

School PE teachers participated in a training programme (4 h of duration) for the implementation of intervention strategies. Training consisted of an exhibition about the current context of health-related physical fitness and body image in adolescence, group dynamics that integrated physical fitness components in a practical way, and from the presentation of the intervention proposal, the role of the PE teacher was highlighted in the intervention and support material was delivered. In addition to training conducted with PE teachers, all school teachers participated in a 90-min meeting to present the aims and activities of the "*MEXA-SE*" programme.

Control Group

Both the IG and CG received the standard school curriculum as determined by the Brazilian government, which allocates 135 min of PE classes per week (3 school sessions). The mandatory PE curriculum was the content of games, sports, dancing, martial arts, and gymnastics. The school activities of the CG remained unchanged. The three weekly 45-min PE classes were conducted by PE teachers at school, following annual planning.

2.3. Variable Measures

CRF, the primary outcome, was assessed using the 20-m SR test using standard procedures [18], validated for Brazilian use [19]. We analysed the following indicators of 20-m SR: Laps; stages; minutes; and maximum oxygen consumption (VO2max), using the equation proposed by Leger et al [18].

Anthropometric measurements were conducted by anthropometrists certified by The International Society for the Advancement of Kinanthropometry [20]. Calculations of technical error of measurement were carried out for all anthropometric measures, which are considered acceptable for experienced evaluators [21] (height: Intra evaluator = 0.28%, inter evaluator = 0.20%; triceps skinfold (TR): Intra evaluator = 1.64%, inter evaluator = 3.91%; and subscapular skinfold (SE): Intra evaluator = 2.64%, inter evaluator = 7.27%).

Overall PA was self-reported using a list of MVPA validated for Brazilian adolescents (ICC = 0.88; CI 95%: 0.84–0.91) [22] and showed a reproducibility Kappa value of 0.45 (89.3% agreement). This list [22] included PA which was organised into different PA types: Collective PA/sports (e.g., soccer, basketball, volleyball, and indoor soccer, in 7 items), individual PA/sports (e.g., swimming, athletics, martial arts, and gymnastic, in 8 items), ride in PA (e.g., skateboarding/rollerblading and cycling, in 2 items), walking (i.e., leisure, transportation, and walking with dog, in 3 items), popular games (e.g., dodgeball and "forty-forty", in 2 items), and strengthening PA (e.g., weight training and abdominal exercises, in 2 items). Students reported the frequency and duration of each daily PA that they performed in the previous week. Thus, we estimated the weekly time (in minutes) of total MVPA.

The time spent in MVPA within school was measured with an Actigraph GT3X+ accelerometer, secured on the right hip by an elastic band around the waist. Wear time was determined by subtracting the time when the accelerometer was given to children (beginning of class) from the time the accelerometer was retrieved (end of class). Students wore the device for four days (from Monday to Thursday) during school time (from 7:30 to 11:30 or from 13:00 to 17:00). We considered valid data using the accelerometer for three or more days and for at least three hours per day. Data were analysed in 15-second epochs [23]. The measure used in this study to characterise the PA at school was the total minutes of MVPA, according to Everson et al [23] cut points.

Socioeconomic status (SES) was measured using a questionnaire [24]. This questionnaire estimates the purchasing power of families and ranks them from richest (A1, A2, B1, B2) to poorest (C1, C2, D, E) based on the accumulation of material goods, housing conditions, number of working individuals in the household, and the education level of the household head. The instrument provides a score for each item according to the amount present in the home and the degree of instruction of the head of the household. Finally, the sum of the scores obtained in all the items makes it possible to classify according to the abovementioned classes (Available online: http://www.abep.org/criterio-brasil). For purposes of analysis, classes A1, A2, B1, B2 were grouped into "A+B", and C1, C2, D, E were grouped into "C+D+E".

Sexual maturation was self-assessed by the participants by classifying their breast (girls) and genital (boys) development in five pubertal stages, as proposed by Tanner [25] and validated at the UFSC (Kendall's correlation coefficient of 0.627 ($p < 0.01$) for boys and 0.739 ($p < 0.01$) for girls) [26]. The students were classified as prepubescent (stage 1), pubescent (stages 2 to 4), and postpubescent (stage 5).

Attendance in PE lessons was registered by the PE teacher in each lesson. This procedure was conducted before the start of activities.

2.4. Data Collection

The data collection team was composed of professors and students of the undergraduate and graduate PE and nutrition courses. Team members received training for the application of questionnaires and for the standardisation of measurements and motor tests. The instruments were applied in the respective order: Questionnaire (first day), anthropometric measurements, 20-m SR test, and sexual maturation (second day). Data collection was performed during students' class period at school. The average duration was 10 days at baseline and at follow-up (Figure 1). It was not possible to blind the staff as to which group the assessed students belonged to because the availability of human resources was limited. It was also not possible to blind students and PE teachers to the allocation due to the intervention characteristics (different activities to those conducted in PE classes before the start of the intervention). The intervention timeline is shown in Figure 1.

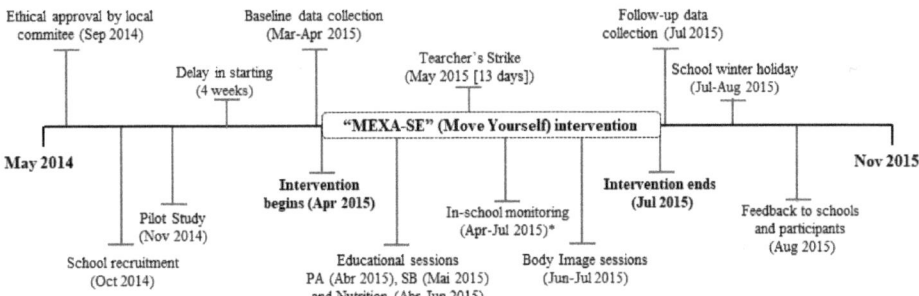

Figure 1. Timeline of the *"MEXA-SE"* intervention study. Note: PA: Physical activity; SB: Sedentary behaviour; *In-school monitoring comprised observations of physical education classes and school recess.

2.5. Statistical Analysis

Means and standard deviations were calculated at baseline and post-test for continuous variables (CRF, age, body mass, height, sum of TR and SE skinfold (TR+SE), PA in school, and overall PA). The normality of data was determined by values of skewness and kurtosis (± 3) [27], confirmed by the display of values and histograms. The height and differences between post- and pre-test for minutes, laps, stages and VO2max showed normal distribution. The variables of body mass, TR+SE, minutes, and laps were transformed by log, VO2max by reciprocal (1/VO2max), and MVPA within school by square root. Chronological age, minutes of practice of overall PA, and stages of sexual maturation did not present normal distribution.

Mean and proportions differences between intervention and control participants at baseline were compared by independent *t* (parametric variables) and Mann–Whitney *U* (nonparametric variables) tests and chi-square analysis, respectively. To determine the effects of the intervention, analysis of covariance (ANCOVA) was used, with the change in CRF as the dependent variable, groups as the independent variable, and baseline data of CRF, sex, age group, SES, sexual maturation, overall PA, MVPA in school, and TR+SE as the covariates. The effect of the intervention was also tested from the intention-to-treat analysis (dropout data imputed by the repetition of the last observation—simple imputation) using analysis of covariance in order to assess the possible impact of sample losses in the intervention effect. In addition, we tested the interaction of all covariates with the intervention effect. We considered the existence of interaction when the p-value < 0.10 [28]. The level of significance for the study was 5% for two-tailed tests using the statistical software SPSS 15.0®(SPSS IBM Inc., Chicago, IL, USA). The effect of the intervention on CRF was calculated for each outcome using the standardised mean difference (SMD) with a 95% confidence interval (95% CI) in Review Manager.

The analyses performed had a statistical power higher than 80% and 5% significance level for two-tailed tests. In the adjusted analysis of variance with group vs. time (baseline and follow-up comparisons, considering a conservative intermeasured correlation of 0.1 (Available online: http://www.gpower.hhu.de/), the ES found was ≥0.10.

2.6. Ethical Considerations

This study was conducted in accordance with the Declaration of Helsinki and it was approved by the Ethics Committee on Human Research of Carmela Dutra Maternity (process No. 780.303). The informed written consent of parents or guardians and the assent of participants were obtained.

3. Results

3.1. Participants

Of 1854 students enrolled in the five biggest schools, 1011 (two schools: 568 in IG and 443 in CG) from 6th to 9th grade (aged 9 to 16 years) were invited to take part. Of these, 568 students provided parental consent and personal assent (60.2% in IG and 51.0% CG). Of 568 participants, 89.8% (IG) and 93.4% (CG) completed baseline measures. In follow-up measures, the response rate was 80.5% and 87.7% in IG and CG, respectively. Considering the time of intervention, the reasons for dropout were absence (10.7%), giving up (7.1%), motor limitation (3.2%), and school change (2.5%). Finally, 432 students (247 in the IG, 185 in the CG) participated in the study at both baseline and follow-up (Figure 2).

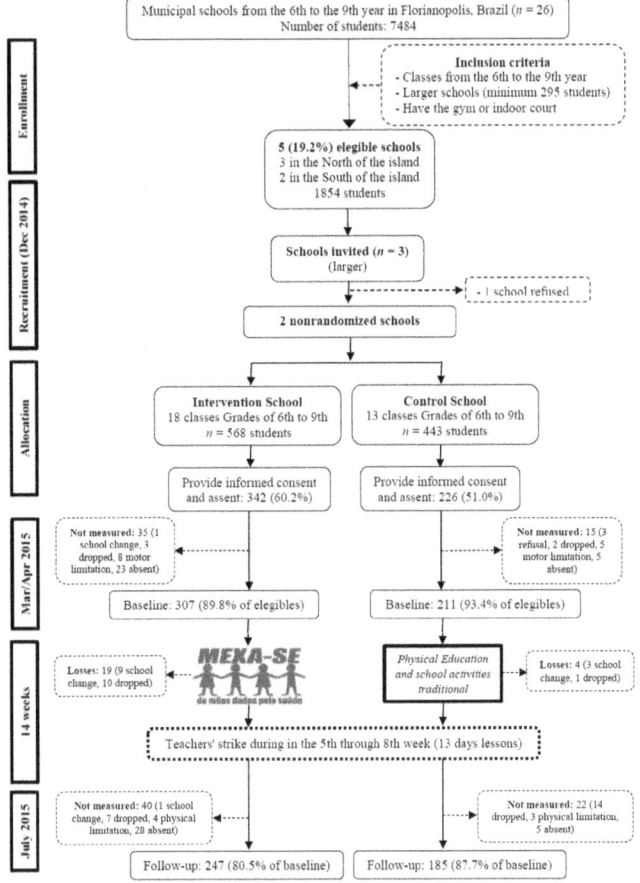

Figure 2. Flowchart of cardiorespiratory fitness. Florianopolis, Brazil, 2015. Mar: March; Apr: April; Dec: December.

Deviations

Deviations from the planned study delayed the onset of intervention by four weeks because of a delay on liberation of schools by the Municipal Department of Education; a teachers' strike from the fifth to the eighth week (13 days of lessons) of intervention also disrupted the schedule. After the delay, the intervention occurred in 11 weeks (Figure 2).

3.2. Comparison of Baseline Characteristics

In baseline measurements, students in the CG had greater mean values for body mass, TR+SE, attendance to PE lessons, and low performance in the CRF test than the IG ($p < 0.05$). Baseline data were also compared between dropouts and students who completed the intervention. Dropouts had greater mean values of body mass and TR+SE, and fewer minutes of MVPA practice, and less attendance of PE lessons. However, there were no differences for age, height, CRF (minutes, laps, stages, and VO2max), sex, SES, and sexual maturation variables (Table 2).

Table 2. Baseline physical and sociodemographic characteristics, and physiological measures in intervention and control groups in Brazilian students. Florianopolis, SC, Brazil, 2015.

Variables	IG (n = 247)	CG (n = 185)	p-value	All (n = 432)	Dropout (n = 136)	p-value
	Mean (sd)	Mean (sd)		Mean (sd)	Mean (sd)	
Age (years) †	12.4 (1.3)	12.7 (1.3)	0.052	12.6 (1.3)	12.8 (1.4)	0.084
Body mass (kg) *	47.7 (11.3)	50.2 (12.4)	0.047	48.8 (11.8)	52.9 (13.4)	0.002
Height (cm) *	155.5 (9.8)	156.6 (9.9)	0.237	156.0 (9.8)	157.8 (9.8)	0.082
TR+SE (mm) *	22.5 (11.5)	24.4 (11.5)	0.042	23.3 (11.6)	26.9 (13.3)	0.004
MVPA school (min)	10.8 (6.6)	10.4 (6.6)	0.499	10.8 (6.6)	10.1 (5.6)	0.833
PA general (min) †	688.6 (913.2)	648.2 (831.3)	0.935	671.0 (877.7)	572.4 (902.6)	0.029
Attendance PE lessons (%) †	83.8 (13.3)	92.0 (8.3)	<0.001	87.3 (12.2)	72.4 (23.4)	<0.001
Minutes *	3.4 (1.8)	3.0 (1.7)	0.009	3.2 (1.8)	2.9 (1.5)	0.093
Laps *	26.4 (16)	22.8 (13.9)	0.013	24.8 (15.2)	21.9 (12.3)	0.077
Stages †	3.8 (1.9)	3.3 (1.7)	0.007	3.6 (1.8)	3.2 (1.5)	0.134
VO2max (mL/(kg·min) *	41.7 (4.8)	40.0 (4.6)	<0.001	41.0 (4.8)	40.0 (4.5)	0.075
	% (n)	% (n)	p-value **	% (n)	% (n)	p-value **
Sex			0.769			0.833
Male	47.4 (117)	45.9 (85)		46.8 (202)	47.8(65)	
Female	52.6 (130)	54.1 (100)		53.2 (230)	52.2 (71)\	
Socioeconomic Status			0.190			0.385
A + B	54.0 (129)	47.5 (86)		51.2 (215)	46.7 (57)	
C + D + E	46.0 (110)	52.5 (95)		48.8 (205)	53.3 (65)	
Sexual maturation††			0.705			0.067
Prepubescent (S1)	1.7 (4)	1.1 (2)		1.4 (6)	1.0 (1)	
Pubescent (S2 to S4)	86.8 (210)	89.4 (160)		87.9 (370)	79.8 (79)	
Postpubescent (S5)	11.6 (28)	9.5 (17)		10.7 (45)	19.2 (19)	

IG: Intervention group; CG: Control group; sd: Standard deviation; TR+SE: Sum of triceps and subscapular skinfold; PA: Physical activity; MVPA: Moderate to vigorous physical activity measured with an accelerometer; m: Metres; kg: Kilogram; mm: Millimetres; VO₂max: Maximum oxygen consumption. S: Stages; † Mann–Whitney test; †† Breasts and genitals; * Independent *t* student test and ** qui-square test.

3.3. Efect of Intervention

The effect size of intervention was 0.15 (CI 95% = −0.04; 0.34). According of CRF indicators (Table 3), the effect size for all indicators was low and not significant ($CI_{minutes}$ 95%: –0.03; 0.35, CI_{laps} 95%: −0.06; 0.32, CI_{stages} 95%: −0.08; 0.30, and CI_{VO2max} 95%: −0.06; 0.33). In all CRF indicators, no significant differences were observed for the IG between baseline and follow-up. For the CG, only VO2max decreased significantly from baseline to follow-up. The results for adjusted differences between the IG and CG and intention-to-treat analysis were not significant. There was no interaction between the groups and sex, age, sexual maturation, and SES.

Table 3. Effect of *"MEXA-SE"* intervention on cardiorespiratory fitness (CRF) among Brazilian students. Florianopolis, SC, Brazil, 2015.

Indicator CRF	Differences between Baseline and Follow-Up				Adjusted Differences between Intervention vs. Control Group					Interaction			
	Intervention (n = 247)	p-value	Control (n = 185)	p-value	Adjusted Difference (n = 432)	p-value	Intention-To-Treat Analysis (n = 518)	p-value	ES	Group vs. Sex	Group vs. Age	Group vs. SM	Group vs. SES
	Mean (CI 95%)		Mean (CI 95%)		Mean (CI 95%)		Mean (CI 95%)			p-value	p-value	p-value	p-value
Minutes	0.05 (−0.10; 0.21)	0.517	−0.11 (−0.28; 0.06)	0.206	0.17 (−0.07; 0.40)	0.173	0.13 (−0.09; 0.34)	0.257	0.13	0.351	0.194	0.558	0.949
Laps	0.67 (−0.58; 1.91)	0.224	−0.83 (−2.24; 0.57)	0.291	1.50 (−0.46; 3.46)	0.134	1.16 (−0.63; 2.95)	0.202	0.16	0.477	0.179	0.759	0.963
Stages	0.07 (−0.09; 0.22)	0.308	−0.06 (−0.23; 0.11)	0.497	0.13 (−0.12; 0.37)	0.307	0.09 (−0.13; 0.31)	0.430	0.11	0.122	0.293	0.894	0.724
VO$_2$max	−0.27 (−0.72; 0.18)	0.240	−0.75 (−1.24; −0.24)	0.004	0.48 (−0.23; 1.19)	0.186	0.40 (−0.26; 1.05)	0.232	0.14	0.107	0.494	0.900	0.882

CI: Confidence interval; VO2max: Maximum oxygen consumption; EF: Effect size adjusted; SM: Sexual maturation; SES: Socioeconomic status; p-value of ANCOVA analysis adjusted by baseline CRF; sex, age group, sum of triceps and subscapular skinfold, sexual maturation, socioeconomic status, physical activity general, time in moderate to vigorous physical activity, and percentage of attendance in PE lessons (Adjustment for multiple comparisons: Bonferroni).

4. Discussion

The results of the current study show that the "*MEXA-SE*" programme had a small but nonsignificant effect on CRF among students. We found a significant reduction in VO_2max from baseline to follow up in the CG, while no significant alteration was seen in the IG. Other indicators of CRF analysed (minutes, laps, stages, and VO2max for IG) did not differ statistically between or within groups. These results are similar to results from a cluster randomised controlled study [29] that evaluated the effect of an intervention targeting the physical and organisational school environment for noncurricular PA (SPACE) on CRF in Danish adolescents (11–14 years, mean: 6m; CI 95%: −20; 31, *p*-value: 0.43).

Conversely, the findings of the current study are contrary to results from a nonrandomised controlled trial [30] conducted during school time in Brazilian students (10 to 15 years old). Intervention strategies were applied in PE classes twice a week for 60 min for one school year; the structure of PE classes comprised 30 min of aerobic exercise, 20 min of playing sports, and 10 min of stretching activities. The results for the nine-minute test were significant for CRF between groups (ES = 0.30; CI 95% = 0.10; 0.50) [30]. The long duration of sessions (60 min) and the length of intervention (one school year) [30] can explain the differences in effect size between studies with the same design (nonrandomised controlled trial) realised in Brazil. Although the weekly frequency of the study conducted in the same country (twice a week) [30] was lower than that of the present study (three times a week), the longer duration of intervention helped to overcome the resistance of the students to the new exercises.

Another reason for our results may be the duration of intervention. The intervention was planned to last 14 weeks, in line with recommendations for promoting change in this outcome [6]. However, this was not possible due to the delay of the start of the intervention (four weeks) and the teachers' strike that stopped lessons for 13 days of the intervention (from the fifth to the eighth week). The teachers' strike in Brazil also interrupted other interventions conducted with students [31]. This external factor is a reality present in Brazilian schools and is a further obstacle in promoting an improvement in physical fitness components. Researchers working in environments such as that found in Brazil should be alert to teachers' strike conditions for future interventions and might be able to mitigate the effect of such issues by planning longer interventions and/or considering the possibility of this type of interruptions. However, we do not consider that this interruption due to the teachers' strike had a meaningful impact on the results of the intervention, as similar results (no significant ES) were found in other multicomponent interventions of a longer duration [32,33].

One of the effective strategies to improve CRF highlighted in literature is the inclusion of aerobic and resistance exercises [6], and higher intensity PA in PE classes [5]. These strategies were included in the "*MEXA-SE*" programme. However, the fact that there is one "free lesson" per week would make it impossible to determine that this strategy is not effective. The PE teacher in the previous year used the "free lesson" system (students can do what they want during class, including staying seated) for all lessons, and with a new class structure, many students were resistant to participation; one of the three PE lessons continued in the "free lesson" system by agreement with students.

In the current study, of the 45 min total in the lesson, the PE teacher needed 15 min to record the presence and outline general content procedure before commuting to the sports field, leaving only 30 min to apply other content. The meta-analysis that aimed to determine the effectiveness of interventions designed to increase the proportion of PE lesson time that students spend in MVPA showed, on average, a 24% relative increase in the amount of lesson time spent in MVPA [34]. The Center for Disease Control and Prevention (CDC) [35] has previously recommended that students should be engaged in MVPA for at least 50% of PE lesson time. This information suggests that pedagogical practice of the "*MEXA-SE*" programme was inefficient and could be improved.

Other intervention designs have shown positive effects on the CRF promotion, particularly those using HIIT [8]. Meta-analysis regarding the utility of HIIT to improve CRF in adolescents evidenced the little heterogeneity ($Q = 9.77$, $I^2 = 28.3\%$, $p = 0.202$), and a large ES ($d = 1.05$, CI 95% 0.36 to 1.75). Ten min of HIIT training has shown to have comparable results to 40 min of moderate aerobic training [8]. Although the evidence of embedding HIIT within the school day is limited, this type of intervention has the potential to improve CRF in adolescent populations [8,36].

The findings from the CG identify that standard PE lessons and other activities did not contribute to improving the CRF of Brazilian students, and a reduction in VO2max was identified in the present study. In addition, attendance in PE lessons was higher for the CG compared to the IG. These results confirm the hypothesis that standard school activities, including PE lessons, do not add sufficient resources to promote and/or maintain CRF in students. Investigations into PE lessons in Brazil showed the reality of exercise in schools, i.e., the reduced mean duration of the lessons (35.6 min, SD = 6.0) and low mean proportion of time spent in MVPA (32.7%, SD = 25.2 or 12.3 min, SD = 9.7) [37]. This directly affects one of main settings to contribute to improvement of physical fitness [6], because for organic adaptations to occur as a result of PA, individuals should be subjected to moderate and/or intense efforts taking place over a certain period [36]. Considering that the only difference between the IG and CG was the exposure to the intervention, another possible explanation for these results is the reduction in CRF that naturally happens with advancing age [38].

There are, of course, some limitations in this study. Firstly, the design was nonrandomised, because school assignment to the intervention group was made intentionally by the local educational authorities. Secondly, we were unable to conduct the study 'double-blind' because the intervention consisted of such a combination of obvious changes and activities that the data collection staff (as well as the students and PE teachers) would certainly be aware of which person or school was in which study condition. Thirdly, the intervention started four weeks later than anticipated and during the intervention period, there was a teachers' strike (May 2015), which resulted in a gap in intervention activities of 13 days. As a consequence, the duration of intervention was 11 weeks rather than the initially planned 14 weeks. Finally, the response rate for post-testing at the IG was lower than expected due to the number of absences of students from school, possibly because data collection took place in the final week of the school semester.

This study was based on the available evidence about interventions on CRF in adolescents around the world [6]. Consequently, it contributes to the advancement of interventions on CRF in LMICs, as Brazil.

5. Conclusions

In conclusion, the "*MEXA-SE*" programme contributed to the maintenance of CRF, compared to a CG where CRF declined in the same period. On the other hand, the lack of changes in the school environment and maintenance of PE classes in the usual model cannot help to maintain this component. The results need to be interpreted with caution due to extraneous factors (e.g., delayed onset of intervention, teachers' strike, and free lessons) that occurred during intervention. This intervention should be retested to show better the real effect on the CRF of the students.

Supplementary Materials: The following are available online at http://www.mdpi.com/2411-5142/4/1/10/s1.

Author Contributions: G.M. and E.L.P. participated in the planning, implementation and supervision stages of the intervention. G.M. analysed the data and drafted the first version of the manuscript, while all other authors (E.L.P., K.S.S. and M.J.D.) participated in the analysis and interpretation of data, as well as critical review of the article. All authors have read and approved the final version of the manuscript and agree with the order of presentation of the authors.

Funding: This research was funded by a grant from National Counsel of Technological and Scientific Development (CNPq), Brazil (process number 474184/2013-7); the Coordination for the Improvement of Higher Education Personnel (CAPES) in providing scholarships to GM (protocol 6674/2015-01).

Acknowledgments: The authors thank the management team: Cilene R. Martins, Juliane Berria, Luiz R.A. Lima, Jéssika A.J. Vieira, André Machado, Márcia C. Simões, and Everson A. Nunes. The authors thank the executing team: Alexsandra S. Bandeira, Amanda M. George, Ana Maria Zofoli, Atanael Rodrigues, Bruno G.G. Costa, Carlos A.S. Alves Junior, Cecília Bertuol, Dominique S. Silveira, Estela A. Monego, Fabiana C. Sherer, Gabriel de Oliveira, Geyson R. Zilch, Jaqueline A. Silva, Lays T. Gripa, Lidiane A. Bevilacqua, Marina S.S. Athayde, Natalia Dias, Marcus V.V. Lopes, Pablo M. Silveira, Priscila C. Martins, Rafaela Castelini, Rodrigo Werlich. We would like to extend thanks to the Municipal Education Department of Florianopolis for authorising the performance of the study; to all members of the school community (managers, teachers, parents and students) of schools involved for the support during the program's implementation; to Mário R. Azevedo Junior, for the technical contributions in the preparation of the booklet for Physical Education teachers and for the exchange of experiences related to the intervention study "Physical Education +"; to the "*Fortaleça sua Saúde*" project for the materials provided, to Danieli V. Rebolho for the elaboration of the "*MEXA-SE*" logo; to Ricardo C. Gomes for the preparation of leaflets and posters, to Ricardo Marcon for the creation of the software to generate individual reports, to Lamartine Teixeira for the donation of office supplies, to the Sports Center of the Federal University of Santa Catarina, and to Ricardo Pacheco for printing of graphic materials.

Conflicts of Interest: The authors declare no conflict of interest.

References

1. Ruiz, J.R.; Castro-Pinero, J.; Espana-Romero, V.; Artero, E.G.; Ortega, F.B.; Cuenca, M.M.; Jimenez-Pavon, D.; Chillon, P.; Girela-Rejon, M.J.; Mora, J.; et al. Field-based fitness assessment in young people: The ALPHA health-related fitness test battery for children and adolescents. *Br. J. Sports Med.* **2011**, *45*, 518–524. [CrossRef] [PubMed]

2. Moreira, C.; Santos, R.; de Farias, J.; Vale, S.; Santos, P.; Soares-Miranda, L.; Marques, A.; Mota, J. Metabolic risk factors, physical activity and physical fitness in azorean adolescents: A cross-sectional study. *BMC Public Health* **2011**, *11*, 214. [CrossRef] [PubMed]

3. Kodama, S.; Saito, K.; Tanaka, S.; Maki, M.; Yachi, Y.; Asumi, M.; Sugawara, A.; Totsuka, K.; Shimano, H.; Ohashi, Y.; et al. Cardiorespiratory fitness as a quantitative predictor of all-cause mortality and cardiovascular events in healthy men and women: A meta-analysis. *JAMA* **2009**, *301*, 2024–2035. [CrossRef] [PubMed]

4. Lee, D.-C.; Artero, E.G.; Sui, X.; Blair, S.N. Mortality trends in the general population: The importance of cardiorespiratory fitness. *J. Psychopharmacol.* **2010**, *24*, 27–35. [CrossRef] [PubMed]

5. Dobbins, M.; Husson, H.; DeCorby, K.; LaRocca, R.L. School-based physical activity programs for promoting physical activity and fitness in children and adolescents aged 6 to 18. *Cochrane Database Syst. Rev.* **2013**, *2*, CD007651. [CrossRef]

6. Minatto, G.; Barbosa Filho, V.C.; Berria, J.; Petroski, E.L. School-Based Interventions to Improve Cardiorespiratory Fitness in Adolescents: Systematic Review with Meta-analysis. *Sports Med.* **2016**, *46*, 1273–1292. [CrossRef] [PubMed]

7. Burns, R.D.; Brusseau, T.A.; Fu, Y. Moderators of School-Based Physical Activity Interventions on Cardiorespiratory Endurance in Primary School-Aged Children: A Meta-Regression. *Int. J. Environ. Res. Public Health* **2018**, *15*, 1764. [CrossRef]

8. Costigan, S.A.; Eather, N.; Plotnikoff, R.C.; Taaffe, D.R.; Lubans, D.R. High-intensity interval training for improving health-related fitness in adolescents: A systematic review and meta-analysis. *Br. J. Sports Med.* **2015**, *49*, 1253–1261. [CrossRef]

9. Brasil. Instituto Brasileiro de Geografia e Estatística (IBGE). Informação Demográfica e Socioeconômica Número 28. Indicadores Sociais Municipais. Uma Análise dos Resultados do Censo Demográfico 2010. Rio de Janeiro: IBGE. 2010. Available online: http://ibge.gov.br/home/estatistica/populacao/condicaodevida/pof/2008_2009 (accessed on 21 January 2016).

10. Brasil. Presidente da República. Decreto Nº 6.286, de 5 de dezembro de 2007. Institui o Programa Saúde na Escola (PSE), e dá Outras Providências. Diário Oficial da União, P.E., Brasília, DF, 5 dez., Ed. Available online: http://www.planalto.gov.br/ccivil_03/_ato2007-2010/2007/decreto/d6286.htm (accessed on 29 June 2014).

11. Bandura, A. Health promotion by social cognitive means. *Health Educ. Behav.* **2004**, *31*, 143–164. [CrossRef]

12. Bronfenbrenner, B. *Ecological Models of Human Development*; Elsevier: Oxford, UK, 1994.

13. Seefeldt, V.; Malina, R.M.; Clark, M.A. Factors affecting levels of physical activity in adults. *Sports Med.* **2002**, *32*, 143–168. [CrossRef]

14. Stotz, E.N. Enfoques sobre educação e saúde. In *Participação Popular, Educação e Saúde: Teoria e Prática*; Valla, V.V., Stotz, E.N., Eds.; Relume-Dumará: Rio de Janeiro, Brazil, 2003; pp. 11–22.

15. United States Department of Health and Human Services (USDHHS). *Physical Activity Evaluation Handbook*; Department of Health and Human Services, Ed.; Centers for Disease Control and Prevention: Atlanta, GA, USA, 2002.

16. Prefeitura Municipal de Florianopolis. Secretaria Minicipal de Educação. Departamento de Educação Fundamental. Proposta Curricular. Florianópolis, 2008. Available online: http://www.pmf.sc.gov.br/arquivos/arquivos/pdf/09_04_2018_14.01.14.62a2765c21e81be772971fd729542791.pdf (accessed on 12 June 2014).

17. Brasil; Secretaria de Educação Fundamental. *Parâmetros Curriculares Nacionais: Educação Física*; MEC/SEF: Brasília, Brazil, 1998; p. 114. Available online: http://portal.mec.gov.br/seb/arquivos/pdf/livro07.pdf (accessed on 10 September 2013).

18. Leger, L.A.; Mercier, D.; Gadoury, C.; Lambert, J. The multistage 20 metre shuttle run test for aerobic fitness. *J. Sports Sci.* **1988**, *6*, 93–101. [CrossRef] [PubMed]

19. Duarte, M.F.S.; Duarte, C.R. Validade do teste aeróbico de corrida de vai-e-vem de 20 metros. *Rev. Bras. Cienc. Mov.* **2001**, *9*, 7–14.

20. Stewart-Brown, S. What Is the Evidence on School Health Promotion in Improving Health or Preventing Disease and, Specifically, What Is the Effectiveness of the Health Promoting Schools Approach? *WHO Regional Office for Europe: Copenhagen*. Available online: http://www.euro.who.int/document/e88185.pdf (accessed on 5 July 2006).

21. Gore, C.; Norton, K.; Olds, T.; Whittingham, N.; Birchall, K.; Clough, M.; Dickerson, B.; Downie, L. Certificação em antropometria: Um modelo Australiano. In *Antropométrica*; Norton, K., Olds, T., Eds.; Artmed: Porto Alegre, Brazil, 2005; pp. 375–388.

22. Farias Júnior, J.C.; Lopes, A.S.; Mota, J.; Santos, M.P.; Ribeiro, J.C.; Hallal, P.C. Validade e reprodutibilidade de um questionário para medida de atividade física em adolescentes: Uma adaptação do Self-Administered Physical Activity Checklist. *Rev. Bras. Epidemiol.* **2012**, *15*, 198–210. [CrossRef]

23. Evenson, K.R.; Catellier, D.J.; Gill, K.; Ondrak, K.S.; McMurray, R.G. Calibration of two objective measures of physical activity for children. *J. Sports Sci.* **2008**, *26*, 1557–1565. [CrossRef]

24. Brasil. Associação Brasileira de Empresas de Pesquisa (ABEP). *Critério de Classificação Econômica Brasil.* 2012. Available online: http://www.abep.org/new/criterioBrasil.aspx (accessed on 5 March 2014).

25. Tanner, N.G. *Growth at Adolescence*; Blackwell Scientificm Publications: Oxford, UK, 1962.

26. Adami, F.; Vasconcelos, F.D.A.G.D. Obesidade e maturação sexual precoce em escolares de Florianópolis—SC. *Rev. Bras. Epidemiol.* **2008**, *11*, 549–560. [CrossRef]

27. George, D.; Mallery, P. SPSS for Windows Step by Step: A Simple Guide and Reference. 11.0 Update. Available online: http://wps.ablongman.com/wps/media/objects/385/394732/george4answers.pdf (accessed on 8 January 2019).

28. Lubans, D.R.; Morgan, P.J.; Callister, R. Potential moderators and mediators of intervention effects in an obesity prevention program for adolescent boys from disadvantaged schools. *J. Sci. Med. Sport* **2012**, *15*, 519–525. [CrossRef] [PubMed]

29. Christiansen, L.B.; Toftager, M.; Boyle, E.; Kristensen, P.L.; Troelsen, J. Effect of a school environment intervention on adolescent adiposity and physical fitness. *Scand. J. Med. Sci. Sports* **2013**, *23*, 381–389. [CrossRef] [PubMed]

30. Farias, E.S.; Carvalho, W.R.G.; Gonçalves, E.M.; Guerra-Júnior, G. Efeito da atividade física programada sobre a aptidão física em escolares adolescentes. *Revista Brasileira Cineantropometria Desempenho Humano* **2010**, *12*, 98–105.

31. Nahas, M.V.; de Barros, M.V.; de Assis, M.A.; Hallal, P.C.; Florindo, A.A.; Konrad, L. Methods and participant characteristics of a randomized intervention to promote physical activity and healthy eating among brazilian high school students: The Saude na Boa project. *J. Phys. Act. Health* **2009**, *6*, 153–162. [CrossRef]

32. Jago, R.; McMurray, R.G.; Drews, K.L.; Moe, E.L.; Murray, T.; Pham, T.H.; Venditti, E.M.; Volpe, S.L. HEALTHY Intervention: Fitness, Physical Activity, and Metabolic Syndrome Results. *Med. Sci. Sports Exerc.* **2011**, *43*, 1513–1522. [CrossRef]

33. Singh, A.S.; Chin A Paw, M.J.M.; Brug, J.; van Mechelen, W. Short-term effects of school-based weight gain prevention among adolescents. *Arch. Pediatr. Adolesc. Med.* **2007**, *161*, 565–571. [CrossRef] [PubMed]

34. Lonsdale, C.; Rosenkranz, R.R.; Peralta, L.R.; Bennie, A.; Fahey, P.; Lubans, D.R. A systematic review and meta-analysis of interventions designed to increase moderate-to-vigorous physical activity in school physical education lessons. *Prev. Med.* **2013**, *56*, 152–161. [CrossRef] [PubMed]

35. Centers for Disease Control and Prevention (CDC). *Comprehensive School Physical Activity Programs: A Guide for Schools*; U.S. Department of Health and Human Services: Atlanta, GA, USA, 2013; pp. 1–65.

36. American Colege of Sports Medicine (ACSM). *Guidelines for Exercise Testing and Prescription*, 9th ed.; Wolters Kluwer Health; Lippincott Willians & Wilkins: Philadelphia, PA, USA, 2014; p. 456.
37. Kremer, M.M.; Reichert, F.F.; Hallal, P.C. Intensidade e duração dos esforços físicos em aulas de Educação Física. *Rev. Saude Publica* **2012**, *46*, 320–326. [CrossRef] [PubMed]
38. Malina, R.M.; Bouchard, C.; Bar-Or, O. *Growth, Maturation and Physical Activity*, 2nd ed.; Human Kinetics Books: Champaign, IL, USA, 2004.

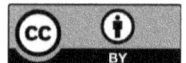

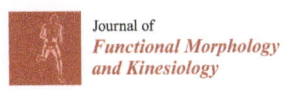

Journal of
*Functional Morphology
and Kinesiology*

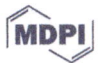

Article

Testing the Motor Competence and Health-Related Variable Conceptual Model: A Path Analysis

Ryan Donald Burns [1,*] and You Fu [2]

1   Department of Health, Kinesiology and Recreation, University of Utah, Salt Lake City, UT 84112, USA
2   School of Community Health Sciences, University of Nevada Reno; Reno, NV 89557, USA; youf@unr.edu
*   Correspondence: ryan.d.burns@utah.edu; Tel.: +1-801-695-5693

Received: 19 October 2018; Accepted: 24 November 2018; Published: 28 November 2018

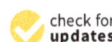

Abstract: The purpose of this study was to empirically test a comprehensive conceptual model linking gross motor skills, school day physical activity and health-related variables in a sample of sixth graders. Participants were a convenience sample of 84 sixth grade students (Mean age = 11.6 ± 0.6 years). Gross motor skills were assessed using the Test of Gross Motor Development-3rd Edition (TGMD-3), school day physical activity was assessed using pedometers, health-related fitness was assessed using Progressive Aerobic Cardiovascular Endurance Run (PACER) laps, perceived competence assessed using a validated questionnaire and the health-related outcome was assessed using Body Mass Index (BMI). The relationship between school day step counts and TGMD-3 scores was mediated through both perceived competence and PACER laps ($p = 0.015$) and the direct path coefficient between TGMD-3 scores and BMI was statistically significant ($b = -0.22$ kg/m^2, $p < 0.001$). Overall there was good model fit with all indices meeting acceptable criteria ($\chi^2 = 3.7$, $p = 0.293$; Root Mean Square Error of Approximation (RMSEA) = 0.062, 90% Confidence Interval (C.I.): 0.00–0.23; Comparative Fit Index (CFI) = 0.98; Tucker-Lewis Index (TLI) = 0.96; Standardized Root Mean Square Residual (SRMR) = 0.052). The comprehensive conceptual model explaining the inter-relationships among motor competence and health-related variables was empirically validated with the relationship between physical activity and gross motor skills mediated through both perceived competence and cardiorespiratory endurance in a sample of sixth graders.

Keywords: anthropometric measures; child motor development; exercise behavior; exercise motivation; health behaviors

1. Introduction

Fundamental gross motor skills associate with children's physical health, wellbeing and performance in activities of daily living [1,2]. Mechanisms for these links include that gross motor skills help children control their bodies, manipulate their environment and form complex skills involved in sports and other recreational activities, which may facilitate optimal growth and development [3]. Fundamental gross motor skills manifest from rudimentary phases of infancy to complicated movements that serve as building blocks for complex movements [4]. A growing body of research shows that these skills may facilitate participation in daily physical activity, which has its own health and wellness benefits [5]. Physical activity has been shown to be influenced by behavioral and psychological determinants across the lifespan [6,7]; gross motor skills may also correlate with these determinants (e.g., independent mobility and active transport). Unfortunately, fundamental motor skills do not develop naturally over time but rather need to be taught and reinforced to the developing child so that they can participate successfully in unstructured and structured physical activity [8].

Stodden et al. [9] proposed a conceptual framework linking improvements in gross motor skills with increases in physical activity in children and adolescents, which will further lead to decreases in cardio-metabolic disease risk. Some of these relationships have been empirically tested and may be partially mediated through health-related fitness [10–14]. The strength of these relationships depends on the current age-related stage of a child's development [15], as the direction of inferred causation is moderated by whether a child is in early, middle, or late childhood [15]. Indeed, much research supports a link between gross motor skills and physical activity and there is evidence that this relationship is bidirectional in nature and is also mediated through the motivational variable of perceived competence [11,14,16].

After proposal of Stodden and colleagues' model [9], research accumulated examining the inter-relationships among the proposed variables. Robinson et al. [17] compiled and elaborated on the mounted evidence in a narrative review linking gross motor skills, physical activity, health-related fitness and health outcomes. The pooled evidence yielded derivation of a similar conceptual model, linking physical activity to gross motor skills via perceived competence and health-related fitness, which in turn relates to a child's weight status. Differences between the aforementioned conceptual models include which construct ultimately associates with a health indicator (e.g., weight status), physical activity or gross motor competence, however it is postulated in both models that these relationships are bidirectional in nature [17]. Research supports pieces of this conceptual model, however testing the model in its entirety has been precluded in the pediatric population. In their narrative review, Robinson and colleagues [17] recommended that researchers should explore the mediating effect of both perceived competence and health-related fitness in the relationship between motor competence and physical activity, explore discrete time periods for physical activity participation (e.g., school hours) and provide specificity in the direction of inferred causation among variables within the conceptual model.

No study to date has empirically tested the motor competence and health-related variable conceptual model in its entirety using a path analytic approach. Doing so will provide the relative strength of the aforementioned relationships, which can help in deriving interventions targeting these constructs. Also, the degree to which the link between gross motor skills and physical activity is mediated through both perceived competence and health-related fitness (e.g., cardiorespiratory endurance) has yet to be quantified and it is unknown whether if there is any residual relationship after accounting for the potential mediators. Even though many of the relationships within the proposed conceptual model are theoretically bidirectional, in the testing of the model in the current study, the physical trait of Body Mass Index (BMI) will be the health-related outcome and the behavior of school day physical activity will be the primary antecedent (predictor) within a fully recursive (unidirectional causative) model. This is because school- and community-based intervention-elicited behavior change is often utilized to positively influence physical traits (e.g., health-outcomes) over time and thus makes the most theoretical sense from the perspective of future intervention research. Testing a comprehensive conceptual model will provide further validation of the model and may spur testing of the models using larger samples of children or adolescents within a specific stage of physical development, which will provide information onto what constructs/variables to target during school and/or community-based interventions. Therefore, the purpose of this study was to test a comprehensive conceptual model linking gross motor skills, physical activity and health-related variables in a sample of sixth graders using path analysis.

2. Materials and Methods

2.1. Participants

According to Kline et al. [18], the minimum adequate sample size for path analyses should be at least 10 times the number of parameters. There are 5 parameters in this study's analysis. Participants were a convenience sample of 84 sixth grade students (Mean age = 11.6 ± 0.6 years; 40 girls, 44 boys) recruited one public Zoom school located in the Western U.S. Zoom schools are given supplemental funding for tutoring, smaller class sizes and extended learning opportunities and the majority of students within these schools have English as their second language. Zoom schools do not have organized physical education classes but have scheduled recess every day for 15 min after lunch. Exclusion criteria were any conditions that precluded students from participating in motor skill and health-related fitness testing. Approximately 67 participants were of Hispanic ethnicity (79.7%), 7 were African American (8.3%), 5 students were Caucasian (5.9%), 3 were Asian American (3.6%) and 2 self-reported as "Other" (2.4%). Participants were recruited from three classrooms. Participants provided written assent and parents or guardians provided written consent prior to data collection. The University of Nevada Reno Institutional Review Board approved the protocols employed in the study (project number: 1018396-4; 30 June 2017).

2.2. Physical Activity Assessment

Physical activity was the exogenous predictor variable with the conceptual model. Physical activity was assessed using school day step counts. School-day step counts were measured using Yamax DigiWalker CW600 pedometers (Yamax Corporation, Tokyo, Japan). Yamax DigiWalker models have been shown to provide an accurate recording of steps [19] and to be a reliable and valid measure of free-living physical activity [20]. The pedometers were worn for one school week (Monday–Friday) between the hours of 8 am and 3 pm. The pedometers were worn at waist level, in line with the right knee. Each pedometer had an identification number taped onto the device that was linked to each participant's name. Data recorded within the spreadsheet included each participant's daily pedometer step count, the average daily step count and specific daily wear time. The unit of analysis was average steps during school time across the 5 school days.

2.3. Perceived Competence Assessment

Perceived competence was a mediator variable within the conceptual model. Perceived Competence was assessed using the Perceived Competence Scale for Children (6 items) [21]. Perceived competence was on a 4 point scale consisting of example statements such as "I could not do better at physical activity" or "I am better at physical activity," with the adolescents indicating on a continuum whether a respective statement is "Sort of true for me" to "Really true for me." Cronbach's alpha for the scale was determined to be acceptable ($\alpha = 0.89$).

2.4. Gross motor Skill Assessment

Gross motor skills was an endogenous variable within the conceptual model. The Test for Gross Motor Development 3rd Edition (TGMD-3) was used to assess gross motor skills. Psychometric properties of the TGMD-3 have been reported with high levels of reliability and validity and is an updated test from the TGMD-2 [22,23]. The TGMD-3 assessed gross motor skills across thirteen movements. Movement skills were assessed across separate locomotor and ball skill subtests. The locomotor subtest items included running, skipping, sliding, galloping, hopping and horizontal jumping. The ball skill subtest items comprised of overhand throwing, underhand throwing, catching, dribbling, kicking, one-hand striking and two-hand striking. Each participant performed the test items across two trials scored based on the respective movement skill's specific performance criteria (0 = did not perform correctly; 1 = performed correctly). The locomotor and ball skill subtest scores were 46 and 54 respectively and the total TGMD-3 scores were out of 100. Motor skill competency was scored using a total gross motor skill score. One member of the research team collected locomotor information at each school and one member of the research team collected ball skill information at each school to maintain testing consistency. Intra-observer and inter-observer reliability were tested on a sixth grade at a different class not recruited for the current study using both live and video scoring. The Intraclass Correlation Coefficient (ICC) = 0.91 for intra-observer agreement and ICC = 0.91 for inter-observer agreement.

2.5. Health-related Fitness Assessment

Two domains of health-related fitness were assessed: body composition and cardiorespiratory endurance. Body mass Index (BMI) was the endogenous outcome variable within the conceptual model. BMI was obtained by dividing weight in kilograms by the square of a participant's height in meters. Height was measured to the nearest 1 cm using a stadiometer (Seca 213; Hanover, MD, USA) and weight was measured to the nearest 0.1 km using a medical scale (BD-590; Tokyo, Japan). Height and weight were collected in a separate room during physical education class. Cardiorespiratory endurance was assessed using the 20-meter Progressive Aerobic Cardiovascular Endurance Run (PACER) that was also administered during physical education class. PACER was a mediator variable within the conceptual model. PACER has been shown to be a reliable and valid test of cardiorespiratory endurance in children [24,25]. PACER was conducted on a marked gym floor with a compact disk providing background music. Each participant was instructed to run across a 20-meter distance within an allotted time frame. The allotted time given to reach the specified distance shortened incrementally as the PACER progressed. If a participant twice failed to reach the other floor marker, the test ended. The final score was recorded in PACER laps.

2.6. Statistical Analysis

Data were screened for outliers using box plots and z-scores (with a ±2.5 z cut-point) and checked for Gaussian distributions using k-density plots. Differences between sexes on all observed variables were examined using paired *t*-tests. Effect sizes were calculated using Cohen's delta (d) with $d < 0.20$ indicating a small effect, $d = 0.50$ indicating a medium effect and $d > 0.80$ indicating a large effect [26]. A path analysis was employed using STATA's "SEM Builder." The lone exogenous variable (variable not affected by others) in the model was school day step counts. Endogenous variables (variables affected by others within the model) consisted of perceived competence, PACER laps, TGMD-3 scores and BMI. Direct relationships examined in the model was the relationship between school day steps and TGMD-3 scores and the relationship between TGMD-3 scores and BMI. Indirect relationships examined in the model included the relationship between school day step counts and TGMD-3 scores mediated through perceived competence and the relationship between school day step counts and TGMD-3 scores mediated through PACER laps. Indirect, direct and total effects were calculated using STATA's "estat teffects" command. Reporting of the results involved communication of the unstandardized and standardized path coefficients. Acceptable overall model fit was indicated by a non-statistically significant chi-squared statistic [27], a Root Mean Square Error of Approximation (RMSEA) < 0.08 [28], a Comparative Fit Index (CFI) > 0.95 [29], a Tucker-Lewis Index (TLI) > 0.95 [27] and a Standardized Root Mean Square Residual (SRMR) < 0.08 [29]. Model fit at the equation-level was also assessed using the multiple correlation coefficient (R) and the coefficient of determination (R^2). Alpha level was set at $p < 0.05$ and all analyses were conducted using STATA v.15.0 statistical software package (College Station, TX, USA).

3. Results

The descriptive statistics are presented in Table 1. Girls had higher BMI compared to boys (mean difference = 3.03 kg/m², $p = 0.023$, $d = 0.57$). However, boys ran more PACER laps (mean difference = 13.1 laps, $p = 0.014$, $d = 0.61$) and had higher ball skill scores (mean difference = 8.5, $p < 0.001$, $d = 1.20$) and TGMD-3 total scores (mean difference = 11.7, $p < 0.001$, $d = 1.11$) compared to girls. There were no statistically significant differences between sexes on age ($p = 0.719$), school day steps ($p = 0.062$), perceived competence ($p = 0.078$), or locomotor skills ($p = 0.061$).

Figure 1 presents the results of the path analysis where both unstandardized and standardized path coefficients are communicated within the path diagram. All path coefficients were statistically significant, except for the direct relationship (direct effect) between school day step counts and TGMD-3 scores ($p = 0.320$). The relationship between school day step counts and TGMD-3 scores was mediated through both perceived competence and PACER laps (indirect effect = 0.001, 95% C.I.: 0.0002–0.0023, $p = 0.015$). Approximately 60% of the relationship between school day steps and TGMD-3 was mediated through perceived competence and PACER laps. The residual error variances between Perceived Competence and PACER Laps were correlated. There was overall good model fit with all indices meeting the acceptable criteria ($\chi^2 = 3.7$, $p = 0.293$; RMSEA = 0.062, 90% C.I.: 0.00–0.23; CFI = 0.98; TLI = 0.96; SRMR = 0.052). Table 2 presents the statistics related to equation-level goodness-of-fit, which provides information related to the effect size at the equation-level. The equation characterized with the lowest explanatory power was on the perceived competence outcome (7.3% of the variance explained). All other equations were characterized as having similar explanatory power on each respective outcome: TGMD-3 scores (23.3% of the variance explained), PACER laps (24.8% of the variance explained) and BMI (22.2% of the variance explained).

Table 1. Descriptive statistics (means and standard deviations).

	Girls (n = 40)	Boys (n = 44)	Total Sample (n = 84)
BMI (kg/m^2)	23.7 † (5.9)	21.1 (4.3)	22.7 (5.5)
School Steps	3376 (1579)	4214 (1435)	3681 (1577)
PACER Laps	22.0 (19.4)	35.3 † (20.9)	26.4 (19.3)
Perceived Competence	3.0 (0.7)	3.4 (0.6)	3.3 (0.7)
Locomotor Skills	36.1 (5.8)	39.0 (6.3)	37.9 (6.1)
Ball Skills	39.4 (5.2)	48.9 † (6.2)	41.2 (7.2)
TGMD-3 Total Score	74.9 (7.8)	88.1 † (10.9)	80.5 (10.9)

BMI stands for Body Mass Index; PACER stands for the Progressive Aerobic Cardiovascular Endurance Run; TGMD-3 stands for the Test of Gross Motor Development-3rd Edition; bold and † denotes statistical differences between sexes, $p < 0.05$.

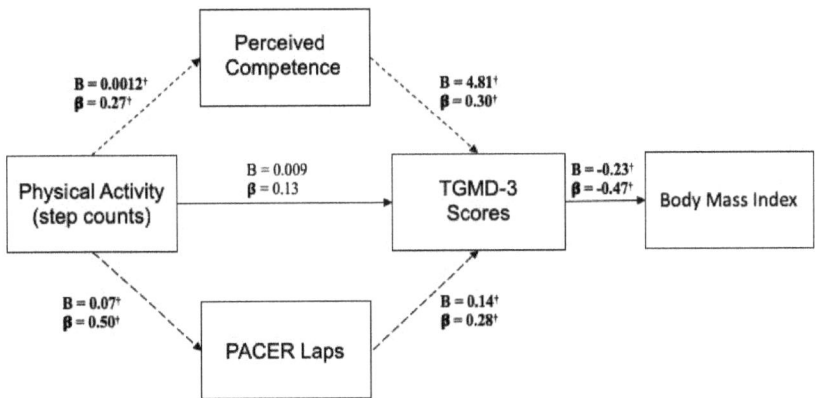

Figure 1. Path diagram aligning with the motor competence and health-related variable conceptual framework. *Note*: PACER stands for the Progressive Aerobic Cardiovascular Endurance Run; TGMD-3 stands for the Test of Gross Motor Development-3rd Edition; B denotes unstandardized coefficients; β denotes standardized coefficients; dashed lines represent a mediated (indirect) relationship; bold lines represent a non-mediated (direct) relationship; bold and † denotes statistical significance, $p < 0.05$.

Table 2. Equation-level goodness-of-fit-statistics.

Outcome Variables	Fitted Variance	Predicted Variance	Residual Variance	R	R^2
Perceived Competence	0.481	0.035	0.446	0.271	0.073
TGMD-3 Scores	119.722	27.880	91.841	0.483	0.233
PACER Laps	457.200	113.483	343.717	0.498	0.248
BMI (kg/m^2)	28.103	6.247	21.857	0.471	0.222

TGMD-3 stands for the Test of Gross Motor Development-3rd Edition; PACER stands for the Progressive Aerobic Cardiovascular Endurance Run; BMI stands for Body Mass Index; R is the multiple correlation coefficient; R^2 is the coefficient of determination.

4. Discussion

The purpose of this study was to test a motor competence and health-related variable conceptual model on a sample of sixth grade students. The results indicated that the relationship between school day step counts and TGMD-3 scores was mediated through perceived competence and PACER laps and the direct relationship between TGMD-3 scores and BMI was statistically significant. The results from this analysis provide information for researchers and practitioners deriving school- and community-based interventions. The results also may direct avenues for additional research exploring other conceptual models. Interpretation of these specific findings are discussed further.

It has been well documented that perceived competence is an important motivational construct that mediates the relationship between physical activity and gross motor competence [9,16,30]. The findings of the current study soundly echo the existing literature. Indeed, the relationship between school day steps and TGMD-3 scores became non-significant without the mediating effect of perceived competence and cardiorespiratory endurance. According to Stodden et al. [9], as compared to younger children, children within the upper elementary and middle school age groups are characterized as having a development period during which perceived competence plays a more important role in mediating the relationship between physical activity and gross motor skills. As a result, it is expected that perceived competence will demonstrate a stronger mediating effect on motor skill competence and physical activity during late childhood than early childhood. This could be possibly illustrated by the mechanism of cognition and peer influence. Specifically, development of growing children's cognitive capacity leads to the comparison between themselves to their peers during physical education class and consequently perceived competence more closely influences their actual motor skill competence [31]. Therefore, children with higher perceived competence are more active and more physically fit than those with low perceived competence [32,33]. In this study, school day physical activity explained 7.3% of the variance in children's perceived competence and the coefficient was lower than a previous study by Davison, Downs and Birch [34], who reported that children's perceived competence shared 27% of the variance with physical activity using a similar path analysis. Several plausible reasons may account for the differences, first of all, the participants in Davidson et al. [34] were girls, while the current study was conducted in both sexes in a co-educational setting. Additionally, the present study employed TGMD-3 and pedometers to objectively measure participants' gross motor skill and physical activity, respectively. Davidson et al. [32] did not test participants' actual motor skill competence and physical activity was assessed using self-reported method, which may manifest limitations in exploring the relationship, as Stodden et al. [9] has concluded that mediating effect of perceived competence on physical activity in middle to late childhood is largely based on the actual level of gross motor skills.

Stronger relationships within the tested model were observed between cardiorespiratory endurance (i.e., PACER laps) and TGMD-3 scores and between TGMD-3 scores and BMI. Cardiorespiratory endurance and body composition (using the BMI proxy) are two domains of health-related fitness. However, in both Stodden et al. [9] and Robinson et al. [17], weight status is an outcome within each conceptual model. The latter model postulates and the current study supports, that physical activity, cardiorespiratory endurance, gross motor skills and body composition are linked serially within a recursive path model. The relationship between physical activity and gross motor skills has been supported in the past [35], however this is the first study to establish that both perceived competence and cardiorespiratory endurance are mediators of effect. According to the observed results, higher levels of school day physical activity will increase cardiorespiratory endurance levels, which will further link to higher levels of gross motor skills and ultimately lower BMI. As stated previously, gross motor development does not naturally develop but needs to be taught and repetitively practiced and executed in order to be sufficiently developed [9]. Improving cardiorespiratory endurance may be a key component in this strategy. It may be that a sufficient level of fitness is needed for a child to be involved in activities that facilitate gross motor skill development. Children and adolescents with lower levels of cardiorespiratory endurance may not be able to participate in the activities needed to optimally develop gross motor skills or they may not spend long durations within activities that foster development of both locomotor and ball skills. Therefore, in order for a child to improve gross motor skills, higher levels of physical activity will need to both improve perceived competence and levels of cardiorespiratory endurance. Without this mediated path, there seems to be no relationship between physical activity and gross motor skill constructs in sixth graders, which emphasizes the importance of targeting perceived competence and cardiorespiratory endurance during specific school- or community-based interventions.

The final link within the conceptual model is the relationship between gross motor skills and BMI. This relationship was quite strong using the current study's sample as 22% of the variance in BMI was explained by TGMD-3 scores. Like physical activity, the relationship between gross motor skills and weight status/BMI has been studied extensively. What is in question is the relative magnitude of the relationship during specific age-related periods of child development and the specific direction of inferred causation. D'Hondt et al. [36] found that weight status and gross motor skill scores were bidirectionally related within two separate mediation models, suggesting that children's weight status negatively affects future gross motor skills and vice-versa. Drenowatz [37] suggests that a focus on motor competence can be used as a strategy for weight management in youth, stating that gross motor skills facilitate sustained physical activity, which over time will attenuate risk of overweight and obesity. Cheng et al. [38] found that higher BMI at age 5 predicted declines in gross motor competency from ages 5 to 10 years old. Although, it is suggested by Robinson and colleagues [17] that the relationship between these two constructs is indeed bidirectional, TGMD-3 scores and BMI were significantly related using the latter (BMI) as the outcome in the current sample of sixth graders. This relationship was direct with no testing of mediation or potential bidirectionality. Mechanisms for this significant relationship could be similar to those similar to that discussed in Drenowatz [37], although Barnett et al. [39] concluded that weight status had differential associations with aspects of gross motor competence. Barnett et al. [39], found that higher BMI was negatively correlated with motor coordination, stability and skill composite but not with object control after a systematic review of literature. This is in accordance with other work where variability in BMI is associated with aspects of gross motor skills characterized by movement in body mass (e.g., locomotor skills) [40,41]. Mediators of effect could play a role in this relationship and given the bidirectionally of the relationships within the conceptual model, it could be that physical activity and domains of health-related fitness again play a role within this potential causal pathway.

The results from this study yield avenues for future research. The relationship between school day physical activity and gross motor skills was mediated through perceived competence and PACER, therefore these constructs should be a target within physical activity programs that aim to improve gross motor skills. Studies have targeted perceived competence in the past when trying to elicit improvements in gross motor skills [11,39,42] however, there may be merit in targeting both perceived competence and cardiorespiratory endurance concomitantly. Because of the reciprocal relationship between gross motor skills and physical activity, targeting these mediators may exponentiate improvements in physical activity and gross motor skills within interventions because of a potential spiral for engagement (positive feedback) similar to that presented in Stodden and colleagues' [9] model. In Robinson and colleagues' [17] conceptual model, health-related fitness is identified as broad construct, not a specific domain. Other domains of health-related fitness, such as muscular strength and endurance or flexibility, may provide additional useful information. Also, in Robinson's and colleagues' conceptual model, there is a bidirectional relationship among many variables, therefore, there is merit testing a non-recursive path model using a larger and more diverse sample of children and adolescents, specifically testing reciprocal paths between physical activity and gross motor skills and between gross motor skills and BMI. Finally, as also recommended by Robinson et al. [17], testing the conceptual model during other time periods may provide novel information. School time is only a fraction of the day for many children and adolescents and is constrained by scheduling within the academic classroom; therefore, testing the relationships within the model outside of school and/or on the weekends may provide important information that can be used for future interventions.

There are limitations to this study that must be considered before the results can be generalized. First, the study sample consisted of students recruited from one school from the western U.S. characterized by distinct ethnic/racial representation; therefore, the results may not generalize to other geographical regions or to samples with different ethnic/racial characteristics. Second, the study design was cross-sectional; therefore, no causal inferences can be made. Third, only school day physical activity was assessed. The results may have differed if step counts were measured across the entire day. Fourth, the physical activity construct was assessed using pedometers. The construct validity may have been stronger if accelerometers were used to assess physical activity. Fifth, health-related fitness (cardiorespiratory endurance) was assessed using a field test. The construct validity of the health-related fitness construct may have been stronger if aerobic capacity was more directly measured in lab settings (i.e., measured $VO_{2\ Peak}$). Finally, sample size precluded testing a non-recursive model with reciprocal (bidirectional) relationships.

5. Conclusions

In conclusion, the motor competence and health-related variable model proposed by Robinson and colleagues [17] was validated in a sample of sixth graders. The model displayed acceptable fit and most path coefficients were significant within the tested model. The relationship between school day physical activity and gross motor skills was mediated through perceived competence and cardiorespiratory endurance; no significant direct relationship between the two constructs was observed. Results of the analysis suggest that the mediators between physical activity and gross motor skills may play a significant role in gross motor development. Ultimately, sixth graders with higher levels of gross motor skills had lower BMI, which may improve health risk if tracked through adolescence and into adulthood. Future research should validate the proposed model in larger and more diverse samples of children and adolescents using non-recursive models and also consider individual variability. Additionally, testing other domains of health-related fitness (e.g., muscular strength and endurance) may have merit and provide additional important information within the conceptual model. The conceptual model proposed by Robinson and colleagues [17] was validated in a sample of sixth graders and supports the important link among physical activity, gross motor outcomes and health in the pediatric population.

Author Contributions: Conceptualization, R.B., Y.F.; methodology, R.B.; data collection, Y.F.; formal analysis, R.B.; investigation, R.B., Y.F.; resources, Y.F.; data curation, R.B., Y.F.; writing—original draft preparation, R.B., Y.F.; writing—review and editing, R.B., Y.F.

Funding: This research received no external funding.

Acknowledgments: The authors would like to thank the students who participated in this study.

Conflicts of Interest: The authors declare no conflict of interest.

References

1. Cools, W.; DeMartelaer, K.; Samaey, C.; Andries, C. Movement skill assessment of typically developing preschool children: A review of seven movement skill assessment tools. *J. Sports Sci. Med.* **2009**, *8*, 154–168. [PubMed]
2. Deflandre, A.; Lorant, J.; Gavarry, O.; Falgairette, G. Determinants of physical activity and physical and sports activities in French school children. *Percept. Mot. Skills* **2001**, *92*, 399–411. [CrossRef] [PubMed]
3. Davis, W.E.; Burton, A.W. Ecological task analysis: Translating movement behavior theory into practice. *Adapt. Phys. Act. Q.* **1991**, *8*, 154–177. [CrossRef]
4. Burton, A.W.; Miller, D.E. *Movement Skill Assessment*; Human Kinetics: Champaign, IL, USA, 1998.
5. Sheldrick, M.P.R.; Tyler, R.; Mackintosh, K.A.; Stratton, G. Relationship between sedentary time, physical activity and multiple lifestyle factors in children. *J. Funct. Morphol. Kinesiol.* **2018**, *3*, 15. [CrossRef]
6. Condello, G.; Puggina, A.; Aleksovska, K.; Buck, C.; Burns, C.; Cardon, G.; Carlin, A.; Simon, C.; Ciarapica, D.; Coppinger, T.; et al. Behavioral determinants of physical activity across the life course: A "Determinants of

Diet and Physical Activity" (DEDIPAC) umbrella systematic literature review. *Int. J. Behav. Nutr. Phys. Act.* **2017**, *14*, 58. [CrossRef] [PubMed]

7.   Cortis, C.; Puggina, A.; Pesce, C.; Aleksovska, K.; Buck, C.; Burns, C.; Cardon, G.; Carlin, A.; Simon, C.; Ciarapica, D.; et al. Psychological determinants of physical activity across the life course: A "Determinants of Diet and Physical Activity" (DEDIPAC) umbrella systematic literature review. *PLoS ONE* **2017**, *12*, e0182709. [CrossRef] [PubMed]

8.   Morgan, P.J.; Barnett, L.M.; Cliff, D.P.; Okely, A.D.; Scott, H.A.; Cohen, K.E.; Lubans, D.R. Fundamental movement skill interventions in youth: A systematic review and meta-analysis. *Pediatrics* **2013**, *132*, 1361–1383. [CrossRef] [PubMed]

9.   Stodden, D.F.; Goodway, J.D.; Langendorfer, S.J.; Roberton, M.A.; Rudisill, M.E.; Garcia, C.; Garcia, L.E. A developmental perspective on the role of motor skill competence in physical activity: An emergent relationship. *Quest* **2008**, *60*, 290–306. [CrossRef]

10. Barnett, L.M.; Morgan, P.J.; Van Beurden, E.; Ball, K.; Lubans, D.R. A reverse pathway? Actual and perceived skill proficiency and physical activity. *Med. Sci. Sports Exerc.* **2011**, *43*, 898–904. [CrossRef] [PubMed]

11. Barnett, L.M.; Morgan, P.J.; Van Beurden, E.; Beard, J.R. Perceived sports competence mediates the relationship between childhood motor skill proficiency and adolescent physical activity and fitness: A longitudinal assessment. *Int. J. Behav. Nutr. Phys. Act.* **2008**, *5*, 40. [CrossRef] [PubMed]

12. Burns, R.D.; Brusseau, T.A.; Hannon, J.C. Multivariate associations among health-related fitness, physical activity, and TGMD-3 test items in disadvantaged children from low-income families. *Percept. Mot. Skills* **2017**, *124*, 86–104. [CrossRef] [PubMed]

13. Burns, R.D.; Brusseau, T.A.; Fu, Y.; Hannon, J.C. Gross motor skills and cardio-metabolic risk in children: A mediation analysis. *Med. Sci. Sports Exerc.* **2017**, *49*, 746–751. [CrossRef] [PubMed]

14. De Meester, A.; Stodden, D.; Brian, A.; True, L.; Cardon, G.; Tallir, I.; Haerens, L. Associations among elementary school children's actual motor competence, perceived motor competence, physical activity and BMI: A cross-sectional study. *PLoS ONE* **2016**, *11*, e0164600. [CrossRef] [PubMed]

15. Stodden, D.F.; Gao, Z.; Goodway, J.D.; Langendorfer, S.J. Dynamic relationships between motor skill competence and health-related fitness in youth. *Pediatr. Exerc. Sci.* **2014**, *26*, 231–241. [CrossRef] [PubMed]

16. Fu, Y.; Burns, R.D. Gross motor skills and school day physical activity: Mediating effect of perceived competence. *J. Mot. Learn. Dev.* **2018**. [CrossRef]

17. Robinson, L.E.; Stodden, D.F.; Barnett, L.M.; Lopes, V.P.; Logan, S.W.; Rodrigues, L.P.; D'Hondt, E. Motor competence and its effect on positive developmental trajectories of health. *Sports Med.* **2015**, *45*, 1273–1284. [CrossRef] [PubMed]

18. Kline, R.B. *Principles and Practice of Structural Equation Modeling*; The Guilford Press: New York, NY, USA, 1998.

19. Crouter, S.E.; Schneider, P.L.; Karabulut, M.; Bassett, D.R. Validity of 10 electronic pedometers for measuring steps, distance, and energy cost. *Med. Sci. Sports Exerc.* **2003**, *35*, 1455–1460. [CrossRef] [PubMed]

20. Schneider, P.L.; Crouter, S.E.; Lukajic, O.; Bassett, D.R. Accuracy and reliability of 10 pedometers for measuring steps over a 400-m walk. *Med. Sci. Sports Exerc.* **2003**, *35*, 1770–1784. [CrossRef] [PubMed]

21. Harter, S. Effectance motivation reconsidered. Toward a developmental model. *Hum. Dev.* **1978**, *21*, 34–64. [CrossRef]

22. Estevan, I.; Molina-García, J.; Queralt, A.; Álvarez, O.; Castillo, I.; Barnett, L. Validity and Reliability of the Spanish Version of the Test of Gross Motor Development–3. *J. Mot. Learn. Dev.* **2017**, *5*, 69–81. [CrossRef]

23. Webster, E.K.; Ulrich, D.A. Evaluation of the psychometric properties of the Test of Gross Motor Development-Third Edition. *J. Mot. Learn. Dev.* **2017**, *5*, 45–58. [CrossRef]

24. Cohen, J. *Statistical Power Analysis for the Behavioral Sciences*; L. Erlbaum Associates: Hillsdale, NJ, USA, 1998.

25. Mayorga-Vega, D.; Aguilar-Soto, P.; Viciana, J. Criterion-related validity of the 20-M shuttle run test for estimating cardiorespiratory fitness: A meta-analysis. *J. Sports Sci. Med.* **2015**, *14*, 536–547. [PubMed]

26. Beets, M.W.; Pitetti, K.H. Criterion-refenced reliability and equivalency between the PACER and 1-Mile Run/Walk for high school students. *J. Phys. Act. Health* **2006**, *3*, S21–S33. [CrossRef]

27. Barrett, P. Structural Equation Modelling: Adjudging Model Fit. *Pers. Individ. Differ.* **2007**, *42*, 815–824. [CrossRef]

28. MacCallum, R.C.; Browne, M.W.; Sugawara, H.M. Power analysis and determination of sample size for covariance structure modeling. *Psychol. Methods* **1996**, *1*, 130–149. [CrossRef]

29. Hu, L.; Bentler, P.M. Cutoff criteria for fit indexes in covariance structure analysis: Conventional criteria versus new alternatives. *Struct. Equat. Model.* **1999**, *6*, 1–55. [CrossRef]

30. Chen, A. Motor skills matter to physical activity-At least for children. *J. Sport Health Sci.* **2013**, *2*, 58–59. [CrossRef]

31. Harter, S. *The Construction of the Self: A Developmental Perspective*; Guilford Press: New York, NY, USA, 1999.

32. Marsh, H.W. A multidimensional, hierarchical model of self-concept: Theoretical and empirical justification. *Educ. Psychol. Rev.* **1990**, *2*, 77–172. [CrossRef]

33. Wang, C.K.J.; Chatzisarantis, N.L.D.; Spray, C.M.; Biddle, S.J.H. Achievement goal profiles in school physical education: Differences in self-determination, sport ability beliefs, and physical activity. *Br. J. Educ. Psychol.* **2002**, *72*, 433–445. [CrossRef]

34. Davison, K.K.; Downs, D.S.; Birch, L.L. Pathways linking perceived athletic competence and parental support at age 9 years to girls' physical activity at age 11 years. *Res. Q. Exerc. Sport* **2006**, *77*, 23–31. [CrossRef] [PubMed]

35. Logan, S.W.; Webster, E.K.; Getchell, N.; Pfeiffer, K.A.; Robinson, L.E. Relationship between fundamental motor skill competence and physical activity during childhood and adolescence: A systematic review. *Kinesiol. Rev.* **2015**, *4*, 416–426. [CrossRef]

36. D'Hondt, E.; Deforche, B.; Gentier, I.; Verstuyf, J.; Vaeyens, R.; De Bourdeaudhuij, I.; Philippaerts, R.; Lenoir, M. A longitudinal study of gross motor coordination and weight status in children. *Obesity* **2014**, *22*, 1505–1511. [CrossRef] [PubMed]

37. Drenowatz, C. A focus on motor competence as alternative strategy for weight management. *J. Obes. Chronic Dis.* **2017**, *1*, 31–38. [CrossRef]

38. Cheng, J.; East, P.; Blanco, E.; Sim, E.K.; Castillo, M.; Lozoff, B.; Gahagan, S. Obesity leads to declines in motor skills across childhood. *Child Care Health Dev.* **2016**, *42*, 343–350. [CrossRef] [PubMed]

39. Barnett, L.M.; Lai, S.K.; Veldman, S.L.C.; Hardy, L.L.; Cliff, D.P.; Morgan, P.J.; Zask, A.; Lubans, D.R.; Shultz, S.P.; Ridgers, N.D.; et al. Correlates of gross motor competence in children and adolescents: A systematic review and meta-analysis. *Sports Med.* **2016**, *46*, 1663–1688. [CrossRef] [PubMed]

40. Gentier, I.; D'Hondt, E.; Deforche, B.; Augustijn, M.; Hoorne, S.; Verlaecke, K.; De Bourdeaudhuij, I.; Lenoir, M. Fine and gross motor skills differ between healthy-weight and obese children. *Res. Dev. Dis.* **2013**, *34*, 4043–4051. [CrossRef] [PubMed]

41. Robinson, L.E.; Rudsill, M.E.; Goodway, J. Instructional climates in preschool children who are at-risk. Part II: Perceived physical competence. *Res. Q. Exerc. Sport* **2009**, *80*, 543–551. [CrossRef] [PubMed]

42. Robinson, L.E. The relationship between perceived physical competence and fundamental motor skills in preschool children. *Child Care Health Dev.* **2010**, *37*, 589–596. [CrossRef] [PubMed]

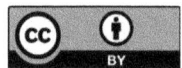

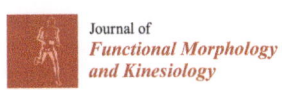

Journal of
*Functional Morphology
and Kinesiology*

Article

Relationships between Motor Competence, Physical Activity, and Obesity in British Preschool Aged Children

Charlotte J. S. Hall, Emma L. J. Eyre, Samuel W. Oxford and Michael J. Duncan *

Centre for Sport, Exercise and Life Sciences, Coventry University, Coventry CV1 5FB, UK;
hallc13@uni.coventry.ac.uk (C.J.S.H.); ab2223@coventry.ac.uk (E.L.J.E.); apx327@coventry.ac.uk (S.W.O.)
* Correspondence: aa8396@coventry.ac.uk

Received: 24 October 2018; Accepted: 19 November 2018; Published: 21 November 2018

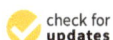

check for
updates

Abstract: Background: This cross-sectional study aimed to examine associations between motor competence, physical activity, and obesity in British children aged three to five years. Method: Motor competence (MC) was assessed using the Test of Gross Motor Development-2. Physical activity (PA) was assessed using triaxial wrist-worn accelerometers. Children were assessed on compliance to current PA recommendations of $\geq$180 min of total PA (TPA) and $\geq$60 min of moderate-to-vigorous PA (MVPA) for health benefits. Associations were explored with Pearson's product moments and weight-status, and sex-differences were explored with independent t-tests and chi-squared analysis. Results: A total of 166 children (55% males; 4.28 $\pm$ 0.74 years) completed MC and PA assessments. Associations were found between PA and MC (TPA and overall MC, TPA and object-control MC (OC), MVPA and overall MC, and MVPA and OC). This study suggests that good motor competence is an important correlate of children meeting physical activity guidelines for health.

Keywords: physical activity; motor competence; preschool; children; obesity; MVPA

---

1. Introduction

Childhood obesity is a serious public health challenge of the 21st century, with enduring adverse consequences for health outcomes. Over 42 million under-fives are estimated to be overweight or obese [1,2], and current predictions are 70 million children will be overweight or obese by 2025 [1]. Elevated body mass index (BMI) is a major risk factor for non-communicable diseases such as cardiovascular disease, diabetes, and some cancers [2]. Overweight children have an increased risk of adulthood obesity, premature death, and disabilities in adulthood, resulting in prevention of childhood obesity being considered as a public health priority [2–4].

Overweight children are less physically active than their healthy weight peers [5], and therefore improving participation in physical activity (PA) is seen as a key preventative focus [6]. Current physical activity (PA) guidelines [2,7] recommend children under 4 years complete $\geq$180 min of total PA, including light and moderate-to-vigorous PA (MVPA) (total PA, TPA), and children aged 4–17 years complete $\geq$60 min MVPA per day. In children, MVPA has been shown to play a key role in health, particularly when related to weight-status [8,9]. However, it is widely reported that children under five years are not sufficiently active [8,10–13].

Studies in American and German children using uniaxial accelerometry have reported that children are not meeting either PA guidelines [10,11]. British preschoolers have similarly been reported to not meet current PA guidelines, although weight status is reported to not influence the amount of PA undertaken by preschoolers [8,12,13]. Prior work has reported that British preschoolers achieved on average 38.6 min of MVPA and 96.7 min of TPA per day [8]. In two related studies, examining preschoolers from the same geographical area as O'Dwyer et al. [8], similar magnitudes of PA have been reported [12,13]. No significant sex or weight-status differences between MVPA completion rates were reported in this prior work [8,12,13]. However, the PA cut-points used by O'Dwyer et al. [8,12,13] were validated in American preschool children [14]. Use of cut-points derived from American preschoolers to assess PA in a British population may not fully capture the PA behavior of children, due to the different social and economic environments in which PA takes place in the U.S. compared to the U.K. Conversely, other research has reported that 95.6% of British preschoolers completed TPA recommendations for health. Similar to the aforementioned studies by O'Dwyer et al. [8,12,13], Barber et al. [15] used cut points which were validated in American preschoolers [16] despite investigating children from Bradford [15]. Preschool-based approaches that decrease sedentary behavior and increase PA may aid in combating the epidemic of juvenile obesity. However, to avoid geographical and demographical bias on PA, using British validated PA cut-points designed for British children is crucial to better quantify PA, and would establish valid current PA patterns.

According to Stodden et al. [5], motor competence (MC) is a precursor to PA, and learning to move is necessary for participation in PA. Fundamental motor skills (FMS) develop during childhood, form the foundation for lifelong PA, and are conceptualized as comprising locomotor skills and object-control skills [17]. Locomotor MC (LC) involves proficiency in moving within space, such as running, galloping, skipping, hopping, sliding, and leaping, and object-control MC (OC) involves manipulating objects, to throw, catch, bounce, kick, strike, and roll [18]. There are relatively few studies which report the levels of MC in British preschoolers, although one study has concluded that the levels of MC are low in this population [19].

Despite a dearth of studies examining MC in British preschoolers, other work in Australia has reported that overall preschoolers were not sufficiently active for health, and females are more proficient in LC than males [20]. The aforementioned work [20] also reported that the different aspects of MC were related to PA in differing ways; OC is more strongly associated with MVPA in males, compared to LC, which is more strongly associated with MVPA in females compared to males. For urbanized British preschoolers, overall MC and LC were associated with MVPA, and OC was associated with both MVPA and TPA; males were significantly more active than females, and more proficient in OC [21].

Preschoolers have consistently been identified as undertaking insufficient PA for health [8,10–13]. Associations between PA and MC have been identified in preschoolers [20,21], but establishing current PA levels and the extent to which British preschoolers complete the recommended amount of PA for health with the use of objective and validated measures, and alongside objective MC assessment methods, has yet to be completed. Therefore, the aim of this study was to address this gap and examine the associations between MC and objectively measured PA, and its relationship to weight-status in British preschool aged children.

2. Materials and Methods

2.1. Participants

Following institutional ethics approval (P31810; 16 February, 2015; Ethics Committee Coventry University), informed parental consent, and child assent, a convenience sample of 177 healthy preschool aged participants (males 54.1%; 4.28 ± 0.74 years) from state funded childcare provisions within the Coventry and Warwickshire area was recruited. Schools and preschools that were recruited were from varied socio-economic backgrounds and participants all attended school or preschool for a minimum of 15 h week. Data collection occurred in the spring and summer months of the school term during childcare hours. Children were included in the analysis if both MC assessments and PA assessments were completed.

2.2. Procedures

2.2.1. Anthropometric Measures

Body mass (to the nearest 0.1 kg) and stature (to the nearest 0.1 cm) were measured objectively by trained researchers using digital scales (SECA Instruments, Ltd, Hamburg, Germany) and a portable stadiometer (SECA Instruments, Ltd, Hamburg, Germany). Body mass index (BMI, kg/m^2) was calculated, and each child had their weight-status classified as either healthy (HW: 1), or overweight or obese (OW: 2), based on International Obesity Task Force cut-points [22].

2.2.2. Motor Competence

MC was assessed using the Test of Gross Motor Development-2 (TGMD-2) [23]. Six locomotor (run, jump, hop, leap, gallop, and slide) and six object control (catch, throw, kick, bounce, strike, and roll) skills were assessed. Each skill comprised three to five components, and skill mastery on the TGMD-2 requires each component to be present. Video recordings of each skill (Sony video camera, Sony, UK) were edited into single-film clips of individual skills with Quintic Biomechanics analysis software v21 (Quintic Consultancy Ltd, Sutton Coldfield, UK). Children completed the TGMD-2 in either school facilities. Each skill was described and demonstrated once by a researcher, and each child performed each skill twice. During analysis, each skill was marked by its individual components as successful (marked as 1) or unsuccessful (marked as 0), and totaled with both trials to give a total skill score. Scores were summed from two trials to create a total overall raw score (scored 0–96) following the recommended TGMD-2 test administration guidelines [23]. The skills identified as LC and OC were grouped together according to subtest scores (LC scored 0–48; OC scored 0–48) and the summing of these gave an overall MC score. All analyses were completed by two trained researchers. Intra- and inter-reliability was established for MC assessments within 15% of the final data set. Intra-rater reliability across MC, LC, and OC showed 0.95, 0.93, and 0.81 agreement, respectively. Inter-rater reliability showed 0.71, 0.90, and 0.81 agreement across MC, LC, and OC, respectively.

2.2.3. Physical Activity

PA was determined using wrist worn triaxial accelerometry (GENEActiv Activeinsights, Cambridge, UK). Accelerometers were worn for 4 consecutive days on the child's dominant hand [24] during all waking hours, except for water based activities to prevent skin irritation when drying. A sampling frequency of 100Hz was employed with data collected in 1 s epochs. The accelerometer in question has demonstrated acceptable reliability and validity as a PA measure in children [24,25]. Valid wear time was defined as a minimum of four consecutive days with two weekend days, with at least 10 h of data recorded between 6 am and 10 pm. Non-wear time was defined as 20-minute windows of consecutive zero or non-zero counts [26].

PA was classified as sedentary, light, or moderate-to-vigorous in nature using the Roscoe et al. [27] cut-points, as these are the only validated cut-points for British preschool aged children. This data was then used to determine children who did and did not meet the TPA recommendations, the MVPA recommendations, and the combined recommendations of both TPA and MVPA (WHO, 2010). For assessment of TPA ≥180 min a day, MVPA ≥60 min for zero-to-five-year olds is considered appropriate [2,6,7], and children were classified as sufficiently active if this requirement was met.

2.3. Statistical Analysis

Descriptive statistics were calculated by all sex groups and weight-status, and reported as means (± SD). Percentages of children that completed each PA recommendation were calculated, as well as associations between BMI, MC, and PA, which were examined via Pearson's product moments correlations. Sex and weight-status differences in PA and MC were examined by independent t-tests. Chi-squared analysis was used to identify differences in MC between those who did and did not meet

PA recommendations. A series of analysis of covariance (ANCOVA) were conducted to compare MC scores between children who did and did not complete PA recommendations, whilst controlling for BMI. Data was analyzed using IBM SPSS Statistics Version 21 (IBM Corporation, New York, NY, USA), with statistical significance set at $p < 0.05$.

3. Results

3.1. Overview

A total of 94% (n = 166) of the original 177 children completed all MC and PA assessments, and were therefore included in final analysis. Means ($\pm$ SD) are presented, along with descriptive statistics and PA recommendation completion percentages, for all participants, male, female, healthy weight, and overweight children (see Table 1). Males were more active (TPA and MVPA) and were more proficient in OC than females. Overweight children had higher TPA and were more capable in overall MC and LC skills. Males were more likely to complete TPA recommendations, however females were more likely to complete MVPA recommendations. Healthy weight children were more likely to complete TPA, MVPA, and combined PA recommendations.

Table 1. Descriptive values of BMI, Physical Activity, and Motor Competence.

	All n = 166	Males n = 91	Females n = 75	HW n = 146 53% Male	OW n = 20 75% Male
Age (years)	4.28 ± 0.74	4.34 ± 0.74	4.21 ± 0.73	4.27 ± 0.75	4.33 ± 0.64
BMI (kg/m^2)	16.11 ± 1.65	16.27 ± 1.78	15.93 ± 1.47	15.65 ± 1.11	19.09 ± 1.42
TPA (mins)	279.65 ± 118.33	289.95 ± 119.99	266.90 ± 116.00	279.36 ± 116.48	282.07 ± 137.77
MVPA (mins)	238.69 ± 101.87	248.06 ± 104.85	227.10 ± 97.71	239.18 ± 99.74	234.59 ± 122.61
Overall MC (out of 96)	45.73 ± 12.07	45.73 ± 13.01	45.88 ± 10.75	43.46 ± 12.19	44.29 ± 11.59
LC (out of 48)	26.80 ± 7.60	26.10 ± 8.01	27.80 ± 6.95	26.80 ± 7.83	26.82 ± 6.13
OC (out of 48)	18.93 ± 8.30	19.53 ± 9.04	18.08 ± 7.13	19.16 ± 8.15	17.47 ± 9.29
% that complete TPA recommendations	80.30	82.19	77.97	61.69	45.83
% that complete MVPA recommendations	89.39	86.30	93.22	68.83	50.00
% that complete combined PA recommendations	75.76	75.34	76.27	58.44	41.67

Note: MC, motor competence; LC, locomotor motor competence; OC, object-control motor competence; PA, physical activity; TPA, total PA; MVPA, moderate-to-vigorous PA; BMI, body mass index; HW, healthy weight; OW, overweight or obese.

3.2. Associations

Significant associations were found between PA and MC (Table 2). Specifically, between TPA and overall MC (p = 0.001), TPA and OC (p = 0.001), MVPA and overall MC (p = 0.001), and MVPA and OC (p = 0.001).

Table 2. Descriptive values of BMI, PA, and MC.

	BMI	TPA	MVPA	Overall MC	LC	OC
BMI		R = 0.018	R = 0.012	R = −0.043	R = −0.045	R = −0.022
TPA			R = 0.733 **	R = 0.402 **	R = 0.170	R = 0.386 **
MVPA				R = 0.376 **	R = 0.152	R = 0.367 **
Overall MC					R = 0.734 **	R = 0.783 **
LC						R = 0.152
OC						

Note: MC, motor competence; LC, locomotor motor competence; OC, object-control motor competence. ** Correlation is significant at the 0.01 level (2-tailed). * Correlation is significant at the 0.05 level (2-tailed).

3.3. Differences

No significant sex-differences were identified in TPA (p = 0.267), MVPA (p = 0.718), overall MC (p = 0.908), LC (p = 0.221), and OC (p = 0.342). Similarly, there were no significant differences in the number of males compared to females that completed TPA recommendations (p = 0.544), completed MVPA recommendations (p = 0.199), or completed combined PA recommendations (p = 0.901).

There were no significant weight-status differences in TPA (p = 0.936), MVPA (p = 0.886), overall MC (p = 0.599), LC (p = 0.991), and OC (p = 0.438). Additionally, there were no differences in the number of children that completed TPA recommendations (p = 0.836), completed MVPA recommendations (p = 0.636), and completed combined PA recommendations (p = 0.689), between healthy weight and overweight children.

When controlling for BMI, overall MC was significantly higher in children who completed TPA recommendations (p = 0.008), who completed MVPA recommendations (p = 0.014), and who completed combined PA recommendations (p = 0.014), than children who did not (see Table 3). Furthermore, LC was significantly higher in children who completed TPA recommendations (p = 0.050) than those who did not, and OC was significantly higher in children than completed MVPA recommendations (p = 0.003).

Table 3. Mean ($\pm$ SD) MC in children who met and did not meet PA recommendations.

	TPA Recommendations		MVPA Recommendations		Combined PA Recommendations	
	Met	Not Met	Met	Not Met	Met	Not Met
Overall MC	45.99 $\pm$ 11.16 **	38.47 $\pm$ 10.55	45.17 $\pm$ 10.89 *	35.14 $\pm$ 13.98	45.88 $\pm$ 11.20 *	39.20 $\pm$ 10.77
LC	26.70 *$\pm$ 6.86 *	23.37 $\pm$ 7.52	26.00 $\pm$ 7.19	25.86 $\pm$ 6.34	26.65 $\pm$ 6.90	23.70 $\pm$ 7.47
OC	19.29 $\pm$ 8.35	15.11 $\pm$ 9.53	19.17 $\pm$ 8.09 **	9.29 $\pm$ 11.31	19.23 $\pm$ 8.40	15.50 $\pm$ 9.44

Note: MC, motor competence; LC, locomotor competence; OC, object-control competence. ** Correlation is significant at the 0.01 level (2-tailed). * Correlation is significant at the 0.05 level (2-tailed).

4. Discussion

This study examined associations between MC and objectively measured PA, and the relationship to weight-status, in British preschool aged children. Importantly, the current study also examined the proportion of children who completed the recommended levels of total PA and MVPA for health. Within this cohort, 80.30% of children achieved TPA recommendations, 89.39% achieved MVPA recommendations, and 75.76% achieved both PA recommendations. This data suggests that most British preschool children in this sample were sufficiently active for health. In agreement with previous literature, there were no significant sex-differences in TPA, MVPA, or combined PA recommendation compliance [12]. However, it is important to note that males were more likely to complete TPA recommendations and females were more likely to complete MVPA recommendations. There were also no significant weight status differences in PA.

Positive associations between TPA and overall MC, TPA and OC, MVPA and overall MC, and MVPA and OC, were identified consistent with previous literature [5,20,21]. There were no significant sex-differences identified in overall MC, LC, or OC, which is congruent with previous literature [19–21]. The lack of significant sex-differences can be explained by the age and stage of the cohort, as they are in early childhood and MC is yet to mature [5]. Additionally, there were no significant differences in MC between overweight and normal weight children. Stodden et al. [5] suggests that MC is a precursor to PA; as there are no sex or weight-status differences in PA, as expected, MC was similar.

This is the first study to quantify the level of PA undertaken by British preschoolers using PA cut-points validated with British preschool aged children [27]. This is coupled with use of an objective and valid method for assessing MC [23]. This study therefore addresses limitations of prior studies examining the same topic in British preschoolers [8,12,13]. In the current study, children who completed PA (TPA, MVPA, and combined) recommendations for health-related benefits were significantly more proficient in overall MC. Children that achieved ≥180 min of any PA per day had significantly better LC scores than those that did not. Additionally, children that accomplished ≥60 min of MVPA per day had significantly better OC scores. These findings provide a potential strategy for intervention to increase PA in children, and ultimately to reduce childhood obesity. To improve completion of ≥180 min of TPA for health, improving LC may help, and improving OC should improve the completion of ≥60 min of MVPA for health, and vice versa. Given there were no significant sex or weight status differences in the current study, the results presented here suggest that there is no need for interventions to be sex or weight status specific.

The strengths of this study include the use of a sensitive process-orientated measure of MC (TGMD-2) [23], and objective and validated measurement of PA in children aged three to five years. Additionally, the TGMD-2 is a commonly used and investigated MC assessment measure present in a large proportion of MC studies [28]. It focused on three-to-five-year old children, an understudied but possibly significant age group, particularly given the closeness to adiposity rebound in children. With a 93% compliance rate, this study is still not without limitations. The cross-sectional design, which means causality cannot be inferred, may have underestimated PA, as accelerometers were removed during water-based activities, which included swimming; however, the accelerometers used have been identified as a valid method to capture PA [24].

This study found positive associations between PA and MC in British preschoolers. These associations are particularly strong with TPA and overall MC and LC, and MVPA with overall MC and OC. This study suggests that good motor competence is an important correlate of children meeting physical activity guidelines for health. The novel finding is MC was significantly different between children that met PA recommendations for health and children that did not. Overall MC was significantly better in children that completed all PA recommendations (TPA, MVPA, and combined). Children were significantly more proficient in LC if they completed ≥180 min of TPA per day, and OC was significantly better in children that completed ≥60 min of MVPA per day. This finding provides more detailed understanding of the relationship between PA and MC, and can be used in the development of impactful interventions to improve MC and PA in this age group. It is possible that different aspects of MC may be required to promote PA and vice versa, and may be used to encourage an active lifestyle in young children. However, longitudinal research is needed to better understand causal relationships between MC, PA, and weight-status, but the findings from the current study can be used to inform the design of developmentally appropriate interventions targeting PA and MC for effective preventative medicine strategies to be initiated to improve PA and MC, and reduce obesity, in early childhood.

Author Contributions: Conceptualization, C.J.S.H., E.L.J.E., and M.J.D.; Methodology, C.J.S.H., E.L.J.E., S.W.O., and M.J.D.; Formal analysis, C.J.S.H. and M.J.D.; Investigation, C.J.S.H.; Writing—original draft preparation, C.J.S.H.; Writing—review and editing, C.J.S.H., E.L.J.E., S.W.O., and M.J.D.; Supervision, E.L.J.E., S.W.O., and M.J.D.

Funding: This research received no external funding.

Conflicts of Interest: The authors declare no conflict of interest.

References

1. Ng, M.; Fleming, T.; Robinson, M.; Thomson, B.; Graetz, N.; Margono, C.; Mullany, E.C.; Biryukov, S.; Abera, S.F.; et al. Global, regional, and national prevalence of overweight and obesity in children and adults during 1980–2013: A systematic analysis for the Global Burden of Disease Study 2013. *Lancet* **2014**, *384*, 766–781. [CrossRef]
2. World Health Organization. Global Recommendations on Physical Activity for Health. Available online: http://www.who.int/dietphysicalactivity/publications/9789241599979/en/ (accessed on 6 September 2018).
3. Dietz, W.H. Critical periods in childhood for the development of obesity. *Am. J. Clin. Nutr.* **1994**, *59*, 955–959. [CrossRef] [PubMed]

4.   Lobstein, T.; Baur, L.; Uauy, R. Obesity in children and young people: A crisis in public health. *Obes. Rev.* **2004**, *5*, 4–85. [CrossRef] [PubMed]

5.   Stodden, D.F.; Goodway, J.D.; Langendorfer, S.J.; Roberton, M.A.; Rudisill, M.E.; Garcia, C.; Garcia, L.E. A developmental perspective on the role of motor skill competence in physical activity: An emergent relationship. *Quest* **2008**, *60*, 290–306. [CrossRef]

6.   Warburton, D.E.; Nicol, C.W.; Bredin, S.S. Health benefits of physical activity: The evidence. *CMA J.* **2006**, *174*, 801–809. [CrossRef] [PubMed]

7.   Department of Health. Start Active, Stay Active. Available online: https://www.gov.uk/government/ publications/start-active-stay-active-a-report-on-physical-activity-from-the-four-home-countries-chief-medical-officers (accessed on 6 September 2018).

8.   O'Dwyer, M.V.; Foweather, L.; Stratton, G.; Ridgers, N.D. Physical activity in non-overweight and overweight UK preschool children: Preliminary findings and methods of the Active Play Project. *Sci. Spo.* **2011**, *26*, 345–349. [CrossRef]

9.   Fairclough, S.J.; Dumuid, D.; Taylor, S.; Curry, W.; McGrane, B.; Stratton, G.; Maher, C.; Olds, T. Fitness, fatness and the reallocation of time between children's daily movement behaviors: An analysis of compositional data. *Int. J. Behav. Nutr. Phys. Act.* **2017**, *14*, 64. [CrossRef] [PubMed]

10. Janz, K.F.; Letuchy, E.M.; Gilmore, J.M.E.; Burns, T.L.; Torner, J.C.; Willing, M.C.; Levy, S.M. Early physical activity provides sustained bone health benefits later in childhood. *Med. Sci. Sports Exerc.* **2010**, *42*, 1072. [CrossRef] [PubMed]

11. De Bock, F.; Genser, B.; Raat, H.; Fischer, J.E.; Renz-Polster, H. A participatory physical activity intervention in preschools: A cluster randomized controlled trial. *Am. J. Prev. Med.* **2011**, *45*, 64–74. [CrossRef] [PubMed]

12. O'Dwyer, M.V.; Fairclough, S.J.; Ridgers, N.D.; Knowles, Z.R.; Foweather, L.; Stratton, G. Effect of a school-based active play intervention on sedentary time and physical activity in preschool children. *Health Ed. Res.* **2013**, *28*, 931–942. [CrossRef] [PubMed]

13. O'Dwyer, M.; Fairclough, S.J.; Ridgers, N.D.; Knowles, Z.R.; Foweather, L.; Stratton, G. Patterns of objectively measured moderate-to-vigorous physical activity in preschool children. *J. Phys. Act. Health* **2014**, *11*, 1233–1238. [CrossRef] [PubMed]

14. Sirard, J.R.; Trost, S.G.; Pfeiffer, K.A.; Dowda, M.; Pate, R.R. Calibration and evaluation of an objective measure of physical activity in preschool children. *J. Phys. Act. Health* **2004**, *2*, 345–357. [CrossRef]

15. Barber, S.E.; Akhtar, S.; Jackson, C.; Bingham, D.D.; Hewitt, C.; Routen, A.; Richardson, G.; Ainsworth, H.; Moore, H.; Summerbell, C.; et al. Preschoolers in the Playground: A pilot cluster randomized controlled trial of a physical activity intervention for children aged 18 months to 4 years. *Public Health Res.* **2015**, *3*, 326. [CrossRef] [PubMed]

16. Pate, R.R.; Almeida, M.J.; McIver, K.L.; Pfeiffer, K.A.; Dowda, M. Validation and calibration of an accelerometer in preschool children. *Obesity* **2006**, *14*, 2000–2006. [CrossRef] [PubMed]

17. Clark, J.E.; Metcalfe, J.S. *The Mountain of Motor Development: A Metaphor*; Motor Development: Research and Reviews; National Association of Sport and Physical Education: Reston, VA, USA, 2002; Volume 2, pp. 163–190.

18. Haywood, K.M.; Getchell, N. *Life Span. Motor Development.*; Human Kinetics Publishers: Champaign, IL, USA, 2009; Volume 5, pp. 5–52.

19. Foulkes, J.D.; Knowles, Z.; Fairclough, S.J.; Stratton, G.; O'Dwyer, M.; Ridgers, N.D.; Foweather, L. Fundamental movement skills of preschool children in Northwest England. *Percept. Mot. Skills* **2015**, *121*, 260–283. [CrossRef] [PubMed]

20. Cliff, D.P.; Okely, A.D.; Smith, L.M.; McKeen, K. Relationships between fundamental movement skills and objectively measured physical activity in preschool children. *Pediatr. Exerc. Sci.* **2009**, *21*, 436–449. [CrossRef] [PubMed]

21. Foweather, L.; Knowles, Z.; Ridgers, N.D.; O'Dwyer, M.V.; Foulkes, J.D.; Stratton, G. Fundamental movement skills in relation to weekday and weekend physical activity in preschool children. *J. Sci. Med. Sport* **2015**, *18*, 691–696. [CrossRef] [PubMed]

22. Cole, T.J.; Bellizzi, M.C.; Flegal, K.M.; Dietz, W.H. Establishing a standard definition for child overweight and obesity worldwide: International survey. *BMJ* **2000**, *320*, 1240. [CrossRef] [PubMed]

23. Ulrich, D.A. *TGMD 2–Test of Gross Motor Development Examiner's Manual*; PRO-ED: Austin TX, USA, 2000; Volume 2.

24. Esliger, D.W.; Rowlands, A.V.; Hurst, T.L.; Catt, M.; Murray, P.; Eston, R.G. Validation of the GENEA Accelerometer. *Med. Sci. Sports Exerc.* **2011**, *43*, 1085–1093. [CrossRef] [PubMed]
25. Phillips, L.R.; Parfitt, G.; Rowlands, A.V. Calibration of the GENEA accelerometer for assessment of physical activity intensity in children. *J. Sci. Med. Sport* **2013**, *16*, 124–128.
26. Choi, L.; Liu, Z.; Matthews, C.E.; Buchowski, M.S. Validation of accelerometer wear and non-wear time classification algorithm. *Med. Sci. Sports Exerc.* **2011**, *43*, 357. [CrossRef]
27. Roscoe, C.M.; James, R.S.; Duncan, M.J. Calibration of GENEActiv accelerometer wrist cut-points for the assessment of physical activity intensity of preschool aged children. *Eur. J. Pediatr.* **2017**, *176*, 1093–1098. [CrossRef] [PubMed]
28. Klingberg, B.; Schranz, N.; Barnett, L.M.; Booth, V.; Ferrar, K. The feasibility of fundamental movement skill assessments for pre-school aged children. *J. Sports Sci.* **2018**, *7*, 1–9. [CrossRef] [PubMed]

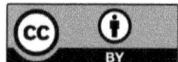

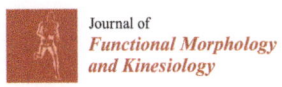
Journal of
Functional Morphology and Kinesiology

Article

Effects of a Sports-Oriented Primary School on Students' Physical Literacy and Cognitive Performance

Yolanda Demetriou [1,*], Joachim Bachner [1], Anne K Reimers [2] and Wiebke Göhner [3]

[1]   Department of Sport and Health Sciences, Technical University of Munich, 80992 Munich, Germany;
      joachim.bachner@tum.de
[2]   Department of Human Movement Science and Health, Chemnitz University of Technology,
      09111 Chemnitz, Germany; anne.reimers@hsw.tu-chemnitz.de
[3]   Katholische Hochschule Freiburg, 79104 Freiburg, Germany; wiebke.goehner@kh-freiburg.de
*   Correspondence: yolanda.demetriou@tum.de; Tel.: +49-89-289-24686

Received: 5 June 2018; Accepted: 23 June 2018; Published: 27 June 2018

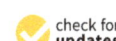
check for
updates

Abstract: As only a small group of children fulfil the guidelines for physical activity, interventions are necessary to promote active lifestyles. We examined the effects of a sports-oriented primary school ($N = 79$) in comparison to a regular primary school ($N = 90$) on students' physical literacy and cognitive performance. To evaluate the implementation of the sports-oriented school curriculum a process evaluation was conducted, in which the school curriculum was analysed and guideline-based interviews were carried out with the schoolteachers and the school director. To measure students' physical literacy and cognitive performance several tests were used. Small positive effects of the sports-oriented primary school on students' physical literacy were shown in standing long jump and attitudes towards physical activity. There were no differences between the groups regarding cognitive performance. This study provides the first insights on how a sports-oriented school can promote students' physical literacy in the future. The results are in line with previous research that shows that when children spend more time in physical education and overall physical activities at school, no negative consequences result for their cognitive performance. In future, long-term evaluations of the effects of sports-oriented schools are required to receive valid results on the effects on students.

Keywords: physical activity; health; students

1. Introduction

In modern societies, chronic diseases represent the most substantial problem in the health system [1]. Systematic reviews show that regular physical activity is associated with positive health effects in children and adolescents [2]. In order to achieve these benefits, children require a minimum amount of regular physical activity of at least 60 min per day [3]. As only a small group of children fulfil the recommended guidelines for physical activity [4,5], interventions are necessary to promote active lifestyles starting from a young age [6].

There are several reasons why schools offer the ideal setting to implement interventions promoting physical activity. First, the central task of school is to improve the cognitive and academic performance of students and at the same time to provide them with the skills and abilities to lead a healthy lifestyle [7]. Second, physical education takes over a major part in the education of the physical through methods to increase physical fitness [8] while at the same time it educates the students through the physical, in terms of physical activities that provide learning, socialization opportunities, and affective outcomes [9,10]. Third, children and adolescents who lead an inactive lifestyle can be exposed to the intervention programmes. Fourth, since students spend a large amount of time at school, in addition to physical education lessons there are widespread opportunities to promote physical activity such as during recess or extracurricular physical activity programmes.

Physical literacy captures the essence of the basic skills children and adolescents should attain in order to be physically active and participate in sports [11,12]. Several models have been developed that try to describe the construct of physical literacy. Whitehead [13] defines physical literacy as "the motivation, confidence, physical competence, knowledge and understanding to maintain physical activity throughout the lifecourse". Based on Lloyd, Colley and Tremblay [11] physical literacy represents the successful interaction of four inter-related core domains: (a) physical fitness (cardiovascular fitness, muscular strength and endurance, flexibility, and coordination); (b) fundamental motor skills (e.g., catching and throwing a ball); (c) physical activity behaviours, and (d) psycho-social/cognitive factors (attitudes, knowledge, and feelings). Numerous studies have shown the importance of these variables for children's and adolescents' health [2]. Overall, physical literacy is a basic requirement to receive lifelong health benefits by being physically active and participating in sports. Against the background of the concept of physical literacy, it becomes clear that the transportation of these core domains is one essential task of school and physical education in order to promote an active and healthy lifestyle.

The question rises whether the promotion of physical literacy comes at the expense of students' cognitive and academic performance. A systematic review suggests that acute bouts of physical activity facilitate children's performance on tests that measure attention, memory, rapid decision making, and planning [14]. Additionally, recent well-designed experiments provide evidence that chronic exercise interventions benefit specific aspects of children's mental functioning [14]. Finally, it can be assumed that the executive skills children acquire during physical education may transfer to academic tasks [15].

In order to promote students' physical literacy, a large number of intervention programmes have been carried out in the school setting [16]. Nevertheless, the effects of these programmes have been small for the most part. Based on these results, it can be assumed that the implementation of temporary intervention programmes is not enough to achieve the abovementioned goals. Rather, intensive programmes spread over the entire school day are promising. Therefore, in this pilot study, we examine the effects of a sports-oriented primary school with a physical activity intensified curriculum and a physical activity-friendly school environment on students' physical literacy and cognitive performance. In a first step, we carried out a process evaluation to develop a better understanding of the implemented curriculum of the sports-oriented school. In a second step, we analysed whether relative to the students of a control school, the students of the sports-oriented primary school would exhibit significantly higher values in the four core domains of physical literacy: (a) physical fitness; (b) fundamental motor skills; (c) physical activity behaviours; and (d) psycho-social/cognitive factors. Additionally, we assumed that the promotion of physical literacy would leave the students' cognition unimpaired or would even enhance it. Accordingly, we predicted that there would be no significant differences in cognitive performance between the students of the two schools.

2. Materials and Methods

2.1. Participants

Participants were recruited from a sports-oriented primary school (intervention group, IG) and a regular primary school without a sports-orientation (control group, CG) in the curriculum. The sports-oriented school is the only primary school in south Germany that provides daily physical education lessons and overall physical activity bouts over the entire school day. To examine the effects of this school type on students' physical literacy and cognitive performance, all students enrolled in the sports-oriented were included in the study. As a comparison, a primary school also located in the south of Germany, in a comparable city regarding size and population, was chosen. Nevertheless, because the control school was larger, a random selection of four out of ten classes existing were included in the study. The study sample consisted of $n = 169$ primary school students (sports-oriented school: $n = 79$; control school: $n = 90$) with a mean age of 8.06 years (SD = 1.21), at the time of the first measurement (see Table 1). Overall, more boys ($n = 101$; 59.8%) than girls participated in the study. One first, one second, one third and one fourth class from each school were included.

Table 1. Numbers of girls and boys participating at the study.

Class	Sports School		Control School	
	Girls	Boys	Girls	Boys
1. Class	$n = 8$	$n = 15$	$n = 14$	$n = 12$
2. Class	$n = 6$	$n = 14$	$n = 12$	$n = 12$
3. Class	$n = 5$	$n = 16$	$n = 10$	$n = 11$
4. Class	$n = 7$	$n = 8$	$n = 6$	$n = 13$
Total	$n = 26$	$n = 53$	$n = 42$	$n = 48$

The sports-oriented primary school is the first private sports-oriented school in Germany. It follows the state curriculum and has been recognised by the German state. The school curriculum comprises daily 90-min physical education lessons active recess opportunities and additionally, the non-sport subjects are taught in an active way. Students in the regular primary school receive three 45-min sessions of physical education. No specific efforts to increase students' physical activity levels during school hours are made.

2.2. Instruments

2.2.1. Process Measures

To evaluate the implementation of the sports-oriented school curriculum a process evaluation was conducted. In the first step, the curriculum of the school was analysed. Additionally, guideline-based interviews were carried out with the school teachers and the school director to gain information about the frequency, duration and content of the physical education lessons, recess and the physical activity during regular classes.

2.2.2. Outcome Measures

The following tests were used to measure the children's values in the four domains of physical literacy and cognitive performance. Because children in the first two grades of school are not yet able to read and write sufficiently, questionnaire items were read to the students and they were asked to give their answer.

To assess physical fitness several tests of the German motor performance test *DMT 6–18* [17,18] were used. This instrument was developed within the scope of the German Society of Sport Science. Altogether, it consists of eight tests that measure students' endurance, strength, speed, coordination and flexibility. For this study, standing long jump (strength; cm jumped), sit-ups (strength; number completed in 40 s), the 6-min-run (endurance; metres run in 6 min), stand-and-reach flexibility (flexibility; reached cm over or under the toes) and backwards balancing on bars with different widths (coordination; 0–8 points) were chosen. In this study, the test-retest reliability of the applied tests over approximately seven months ranged between $r_{tt} = 0.64$ and $r_{tt} = 0.83$.

Student's fundamental motor skills were measured using several tests of the basic motor competences test (*MOBAK-1*) for children in grades one and two [19] and basic motor competences test (*MOBAK-3*) for children in grades three and four [20] test batteries. Each of the batteries contains eight tests differentiating between assessing the ability to move an object or to move oneself. We concentrated on testing skills in moving an object and used the tests throwing, catching, dribbling and bouncing for the children in the first two grades. The older children performed the same tests, only throwing and catching was assessed within one test. The test-retest reliability ranged between $r_{tt} = -0.06$ and $r_{tt} = 0.35$.

Physical activity behaviour was measured with the question "On how many days of last week were you physically active for more than 60 min?" [21,22]. Test-retest reliability was $r_{tt} = 0.28$. Standardised questionnaires were used to measure the psycho-social factors of physical literacy. Students' motivation towards physical education was assessed with a questionnaire based on the *Intrinsic Motivation Inventory* [23]. Their attitudes towards physical education was assessed with the *Attitudes towards physical education* (ESU) questionnaire [24] whereas health-related fitness knowledge was measured with a previously developed questionnaire [25]. Lower values represent higher motivation and attitude. Knowledge is described by the percentage of correct answers. For the motivation scale the internal consistency measured by Cronbach's alpha was 0.62. Internal consistencies for attitudes towards physical education and fitness knowledge were 0.57 and 0.64, respectively.

Cognitive performance was assessed with two computer-based tests: (a) the Simon task in the form of a Dots test [26], which again contains three subtests; and (b) the Flanker test [27]. In a Simon task, a single item is presented in one of two locations (to the left or right of fixation). The participant must indicate the identity of the item with a left or right keypress. Because of the natural tendency to respond in the direction of task-relevant stimuli, response time is faster when the required response (e.g., right keypress) is congruent with the location of the stimulus (e.g., right side of fixation). The Flanker task is widely used to measure interference control. This task calls for the participant to identify a target item defined by its location while ignoring one or more distracting items that flank the target and whose identities may activate the correct (on congruent trials) or incorrect (on incongruent trials) response. For the Dots tests and the Flanker test the inverse efficiency score [28] was calculated, which accounts for speed and accuracy of the students' answers. Additionally, a reaction test was carried out to make sure that differences in performance between intervention group (IG) and control group (CG) are not only based on a difference in reaction speed. Test-retest reliability for the Dots test was by average at 0.69. The respective value for the Flanker test was 0.11 and for the reaction test 0.41.

2.3. Procedure

During the academic year 2014/2015, a pilot study was conducted to examine the effects of a sports-oriented primary school on students' physical literacy and cognitive performance in comparison with students of a regular primary school. In order to receive more reliable results, data were assessed twice. Measurements in both IG and CG took place between December 2014 and July 2015. For the process evaluation of the curriculum of the sports-oriented primary school, teachers and the school director were interviewed.

Information about the study and request for participation were sent to the school directors by the regional council. CG teachers were informed that they were participating in a study examining the development of students' motor and cognitive performance from grade one to four. Students' parents were informed about the study and provided their consent for their children to participate in the programme. All procedures performed in this study were in accordance with the 1964 Declaration of Helsinki and its later amendments. The ethics department of the medical faculty at the University of Tübingen in Germany, the regional council, school directors and teachers approved the implementation of this study (Approval code: 155/16 S; approval date: 12 May 2014).

2.4. Data Analysis

Analyses were performed using SPSS version 23 (IBM, Armonk, NY, USA). Missing values in the scales assessing the psycho-social factors of physical literacy were replaced by the expectation maximization technique. After checking for normal distribution and potential multicollinearity of the variables, multivariate analyses of variance (MANOVA, Sha Tin, HongKong) were conducted to test for differences between the students of the two schools on the examined constructs at the respective time points. The guideline-based interviews were analysed by summarising the teachers' and the director's answers regarding the frequency, duration and content of the physical education lessons, recess and the physical activity during regular classes. Additionally, reasons for not being able to comply with the physical activity aims of the school were listed.

3. Results

3.1. Process Evaluation

Based on the written curriculum provided by the school director, it became clear that the vision of the sports-oriented primary school is to provide students with the opportunities and time to achieve the necessary amounts of daily physical activity and movement skills in order to counter against the health consequences of a sedentary lifestyle. Additionally, the school aims to promote students' cognitive performance through regular physical activity intervals and therefore eventually enhance the students' academic performance.

The structured interviews with the school teachers provided an insight of the elements of the physical activity intensified curriculum and the vision of the school. The broad corridors in the school building provided indoor opportunities for games and physical activities especially on rainy days. On days with good weather, the students spent their time during recess mostly on the schoolyard. Even though the schoolyard provides enough space for movement, the school teachers requested several improvements. For example, they observed that some of the students did not know what to do during recess and therefore did not engage in physically active behaviours. More traditional playground elements such as swings or a slide and a climbing opportunity would be further possibilities to promote physical activity in less active children. Additionally, the organisation of the existing play equipment (balls, skipping ropes) needed further improvement in a way that the students can independently have access to it at any time during the school day.

Eight 45-min physical education lessons were provided in each class over a week including two hours of swimming lessons every Friday. During physical education the teachers set a focus on the promotion of coordinative skills in the first two grades using basic elements such as balancing and swinging elements but also modern elements such as wave boards and roller-skates. In grade three and four, several classical sports were taught such as track and field or soccer.

An important aspect of the sports-oriented school was that the classroom teachers integrated movement elements during regular class hours so that physical activity was not only restricted to physical education and recess. Every morning the school begins with a movement element. For example, one classroom teacher developed a "health box" in which several fitness exercises such as sit-ups, jumping jack, or jump and reach are described. Every morning the children chose five to six exercises that are carried out at the beginning of the first school hour. Another example could be found in lessons teaching foreign languages. While introducing new adjectives, the teachers named several words. Each time the students recognised an adjective they had to stand on their desk. Finally, sedentary behaviour was reduced in class because children were allowed to stand up from their seat whenever they wanted to have a glass of water or to go to the toilet.

The final part of the interview with the teachers addressed the motivation of the students to participate at physical activities during the entire school day. Overall, the teachers emphasised that the majority of the children were always happy to be active. Nonetheless, when a student expressed that he or she was tired, the student was not obliged to participate as long as he or she did not disturb the rest of the class. Few exceptions also existed where some children were never happy to engage in physical activities irrespective of the time of day or whether it was an activity during regular class or physical education.

3.2. Outcome Measures

The comparison analysis between the sports-oriented and the regular primary school is shown in Tables 2 and 3. Concerning the students' physical literacy, small positive effects of the sports-oriented school in comparison to the regular primary school were observed.

Table 2. Means and standard deviations of the two schools at T1 and corresponding between-group results of the respective multivariate analyses of variance (MANOVAs).

Variable	Test	Sports School			Control School			MANOVA		
		Mean	SD	n	Mean	SD	n	F	Sig.	η_p^2
Physical fitness	stand-and-reach flexibility (cm)	0.91	6.93	75	−0.75	6.62	69	2.17	0.14	0.015
	Balance (points)	7.73	4.92	75	6.81	4.35	69	1.41	0.24	0.010
	Standing long jump (cm)	133.60	19.52	75	122.12	21.83	69	11.11	0.001 **,a	0.073
	Sit-ups (number)	16.16	6.90	75	15.49	4.65	69	<1	0.50	0.003
	6 min run (meters)	969.46	157.40	75	928.31	137.78	69	2.77	0.10	0.019
Psycho-social/cognitive factors	Knowledge (% correct)	67.83	20.92	69	71.73	18.89	81	1.44	0.23	0.010
	Attitude	1.87	0.39	69	2.10	0.49	81	9.48	0.002 **,a	0.060
	Motivation	1.61	0.53	69	1.60	0.48	81	<1	0.93	0.000
Cognitive performance	Dots 1	669.41	176.41	69	691.83	237.32	69	<1	0.53	0.003
	Dots 2	844.19	295.14	69	835.47	289.26	69	<1	0.86	0.000
	Dots 3	1424.74	493.90	69	1385.29	896.14	69	<1	0.75	0.001
	Reaction	495.82	128.40	69	461.62	113.44	69	2.75	0.10	0.020

Note: SD = standard deviation; ** $p < 0.01$, a = in favour of the sport school.

Table 3. Means and standard deviations of the two schools at T2 and corresponding between-group results of the respective MANOVAs.

Variable	Test	Sports School			Control School			MANOVA		
		Mean	SD	n	Mean	SD	n	F	Sig.	η_p^2
Physical fitness	stand-and-reach flexibility (cm)	−0.96	7.07	69	0.50	6.96	80	1.67	0.20	0.011
	Balance (points)	7.46	4.35	69	6.19	3.94	80	3.63	0.06	0.024
	Standing long jump (cm)	133.07	21.92	69	123.91	18.68	80	7.59	0.007 **,a	0.049
	Sit-ups (number)	19.28	6.50	69	19.31	5.63	80	<1	0.97	0.000
	6 min run (meters)	1003.01	122.46	69	991.50	133.40	80	<1	0.59	0.002
Psycho-social/cognitive factors	Knowledge (% correct)	78.47	21.07	72	76.05	18.49	86	<1	0.44	0.004
	Attitude	1.68	0.43	72	1.97	0.45	86	17.55	0.000 ***,a	0.101
	Motivation	1.69	0.56	72	1.56	0.54	86	1.94	0.17	0.012
Cognitive performance	Dots 1	640.37	178.17	71	699.68	658.17	78	<1	0.46	0.004
	Dots 2	759.62	254.53	71	735.36	212.00	78	<1	0.53	0.003
	Dots 3	1133.92	349.28	71	1090.64	470.31	78	<1	0.53	0.003
	Reaction	451.12	99.42	71	439.69	87.47	78	<1	0.46	0.004

Note: SD = standard deviation; ** $p < 0.01$, *** $p < 0.001$, a = in favour of the sport school.

Regarding the first core domain of physical literacy, physical fitness, students of the sport-school exhibited significantly higher values in standing long jump at both time points. Group membership explained 7.3% and 4.9% of the variance found in this test at the respective time points. Additionally, there were differences in balancing backwards and 6-min run in favour of the sports-oriented school at both time points, although not reaching statistical significance. For each applied test, the values of our sample were in the range of the reference sample [18].

Regarding psycho-social factors, the students of the sports-oriented primary school showed significantly better values in their attitude towards physical education in comparison to the regular primary school at both time points. Group membership was responsible for 6% and 10.1% of the variance at the respective time points. No significant differences were found for health-related fitness knowledge and their motivation towards physical education between both schools.

The students' values regarding fundamental motor skills and physical activity behaviours could not be assessed reliably. Since acceptable reliabilities build the basis for every scientific examination, it was refrained from analysing the students' performance in the MOBAK tests and their physical activity levels.

Concerning the cognitive performance, no significant between-group differences were found. None of the dots tests discriminated between the groups. Significant differences in reaction speed could neither be found. The values in the Flanker test were not analysed, because test-retest reliability was not satisfying.

4. Discussion

This study is the first in Germany that reported the effects of a sports-oriented primary school on students' physical literacy and cognitive performance and that evaluated the implementation of a sports-oriented primary school curriculum.

The interviews revealed the ambition of the school director and the school teachers to contribute to the achievement of the required daily physical activity levels in the students to obtain positive health outcomes, to promote students' cognitive and academic performances and to improve the students' movement skills. Unfortunately, the effects of the sports-oriented curriculum on physical activity levels could not be analysed within this study, because the reliability of the measure on physical activity was not satisfactory. The interviews further revealed that, from the teachers' point of view, for the successful implementation of a sports-oriented school curriculum that promotes daily physical activity, more than just some additional physical education lessons is needed. Teachers assumed that to foster physical activity during the whole school day encouragement and motivation of students are requisite. The influence of motivational support on physical activity during school days was also demonstrated in interventional studies [29,30].

Furthermore, activity-friendly built environmental structures are needed that facilitate physical activities during the school day in an indoor and outdoor environment, respectively. This is in line with findings from other empirical studies with quantitative designs [31,32] showing that a larger number of outdoor facilities like soccer fields and loose play equipment like skipping ropes at school was associated with higher odds of being physically active in boys and girls.

In summary, to establish an activity-promoting school concept besides a sports-oriented curriculum and supportive social environments (teachers willing to support physical activity during the whole school day) activity-friendly built environmental structures providing space and equipment for physical activities are relevant.

Regarding the quantitative study results, small positive effects in physical literacy can be attributed to the sports-oriented school. In comparison to the control school, the students of the sports-oriented school had significantly higher levels in standing long jump and a more positive attitude towards physical activity at both measurement time points. Furthermore, positive tendencies were observed in the sports-oriented school in comparison to the control school in the 6-min run, balancing backwards and sit-ups (only in T1). Finally, there were no significant between-group differences in motivation towards physical education, fitness knowledge or cognitive performance. Slightly better values of one of the groups were always dependent on subtest and measurement time point. Thus, no indications towards a potentially consistent pattern could be found for these aspects.

The effects of the sports-oriented school on students' physical literacy were small. Based on the information received in the interviews with the school teachers, this could be due to several reasons. It is likely that children from the control school compensated their sedentary behaviour to a great extent in the afternoon hours, whereas students of the sports-oriented school compensated their additional amount of physical activity during school time with a reduction of physical activity during the after-school hours. This is in accordance with the "Activitystat" hypothesis suggesting that the individual's amount of physical activity and energy expenditure is controlled over time to remain constant. Therefore, an individual's increase in physical activity in one setting is accompanied by a compensatory reduction of physical activity in another setting to maintain overall physical activity level [33,34]. Similarly, in a study in Denmark comparing physical activity levels of 1st to 6th grade students from sport and normal schools, no differences in the overall physical activity levels were found. The overall physical activity levels remained stable as the students compensated the additional physical activity during school in the after school hours [35]. Nevertheless, these are only assumptions that need to be systematically examined in future studies.

In our study, there were no negative effects of additional physical education lessons on students' cognitive performance. This is in line with previous studies [35,36], in which no differences existed between the students of the sports-oriented and the regular school in their cognitive performance. Also, in the study by Sallis et al. [37], in which the effects of a two year health-related school physical education programme on standardised academic achievement with 759 children was examined, it was shown that increasing physical education from 32 to 98 or 109 min/week did not reduce academic performance. Despite devoting twice as many minutes per week to physical education as controls, the health-related physical education programme did not interfere with academic achievement. In a recent meta-analytical study it was even shown that curricular physical education programmes even had a positive impact on cognitive functions [38]. Thus, rising concerns that increasing weekly time of physical education could lead to declines in academic performance due to less time remaining for other school subjects were not supported by our or other empirical studies.

Limitations

To the best of our knowledge, in Germany only one school exists that carries out a sports-oriented curriculum including daily physical education and active recess. Therefore, this pilot study is based on a small sample size and lacks the necessary power in the statistical analysis in order to provide solid findings. Nevertheless, this study provides a first glance into the possible effects of a sports-oriented school and gives first indications on positive effects on physical literacy. A longitudinal approach is needed to provide future directions to the development of whole-day sports-oriented schools.

We used generic measurement instruments (*DMT 6–18, MOBAK*) to assess students' physical fitness and motor abilities. *DMT 6–18* revealed high reliability warranting reliable conclusions on physical fitness. In contrast, *MOBAK* showed weak reliability values, and therefore no further conclusions were drawn based on these tests. Physical activity behaviour and psychological determinants were measured with questionnaires. Retest-reliability results of the physical activity behaviour question was very low. A timeframe of five months is very long to receive high reliability values. Nevertheless, values lower than $r_{tt} = 0.40$ do not allow conclusions to be drawn based on the results gained. Therefore, in future studies, besides larger study samples, objective measurements using accelerometers and systematic observation methods are mandatory to capture physical activity levels in primary school children. The reliability values of the tests measuring students' cognitive functioning varied. While the dots test had satisfactory reliability, the flanker revealed very low values and therefore, the results based on this test were not further discussed in this paper.

5. Conclusions

The effects of a sports-oriented primary school on students' physical literacy could only be shown in the standing long jump and the attitudes towards physical activity. Nevertheless, the effects in these tests were small. In respect to cognitive performance, no significant differences between the two schools were observed. This is in line with previous research that showed that when children spent more time in physical education and overall physical activities at school, no negative consequences resulted on their cognitive performance [35–37]. In the future, long-term evaluations of the effects of sports-oriented schools are required to receive valid results on the effects on students. Nevertheless, this pilot study provides first insights on how to improve a sports-oriented school to promote students' physical literacy in the future.

Physical inactivity levels are rising and schools need to adapt their curricula and environments in order to act against this. When also integrating improvements in activity-friendly environments, sports-oriented schools are a promising approach to contribute to higher levels of physical activity and less sedentary time in children during school hours, and to generally promote students' physical literacy. Despite the greater time allocated to physical activity in the sports-oriented

J. Funct. Morphol. Kinesiol. **2018**, *3*, 37

school (daily physical education, active recess), there were no negative consequences on students' cognitive performance.

The results have important implications for school health efforts. Even when it is not possible to allocate daily physical education in the school curriculum, several other low budget opportunities exist to transform the school into a more physical activity friendly environment (e.g., by provision of loose physical activity equipment during recess). The commitment of teachers and school directors is crucial when it comes to the implementation of such activities. It is important that the school directors encourage the school teachers to promote boosts of activities as a first action in the morning, as described by the school teachers of the sports-oriented school. Additionally, a culture of providing the children with more freedom and support to be physically active during regular class, by providing an activity-friendly school environment and loose play equipment, by avoiding sitting rules, and by combining learning with movement elements, seems warranted.

Author Contributions: Conceptualization, Y.D. and W.G.; Methodology, Y.D. and J.B.; Writing-Original Draft Preparation, Y.D. and J.B.; Writing-Review & Editing, W.G., J.B. and A.K.R.; Funding Acquisition, Y.D. and W.G.

Funding: This study was supported by Badischer Sportbund and Spardabank.

Conflicts of Interest: The authors declare no conflict of interest.

References

1. Cecchini, M.; Sassi, F.; Lauer, J.A.; Lee, Y.Y.; Guajardo-Barron, V.; Chisholm, D. Chronic diseases: Chronic diseases and development 3: Tackling of unhealthy diets, physical inactivity, and obesity: Health effects and cost-effectiveness. *Lancet* **2010**, *376*, 1775–1784. [CrossRef]
2. Poitras, V.J.; Gray, C.E.; Borghese, M.M.; Carson, V.; Chaput, J.-P.; Janssen, I.; Katzmarzyk, P.T.; Pate, R.R.; Connor Gorber, S.; Kho, M.E.; et al. Systematic review of the relationships between objectively measured physical activity and health indicators in school-aged children and youth. *Appl. Physiol. Nutr. Metab.* **2016**, *41*, 197–239. [CrossRef] [PubMed]
3. WHO. *Global Recommendations on Physical Activity for Health*; WHO Press: Geneva, Switzerland, 2010.
4. Kalman, M.; Inchley, J.; Sigmundova, D.; Iannotti, R.J.; Tynjälä, J.A.; Hamrik, Z.; Haug, E.; Bucksch, J. Secular trends in moderate-to-vigorous physical activity in 32 countries from 2002 to 2010: A cross-national perspective. *Eur. J. Public Health* **2015**, *25*, 37–40. [CrossRef] [PubMed]
5. Jekauc, D.; Reimers, A.K.; Wagner, M.O.; Woll, A. Prevalence and socio-demographic correlates of the compliance with the physical activity guidelines in children and adolescents in Germany. *BMC Public Health* **2012**, *12*, 714. [CrossRef] [PubMed]
6. Cale, L.; Harris, J. Physical activity promotion interventions, initiatives, resources and contacts. In *Exercise and Young People: Issues, Implications and Initiatives*; Cale, L., Harris, J., Eds.; Palgrave Macmillan: New York, NY, USA, 2005; pp. 232–270.
7. USA Department of Health and Human Services. *Results from the School Health and Policies and Practices Study 2014*; USA Department of Health and Human Services: Atlanta, GA, USA, 2015.
8. Siedentop, D.; Van der Mars, H. *Introduction to Physical Education, Fitness, and Sport*; McGraw-Hill: New York, NY, USA, 2004.
9. Rice, E.A.; Hutchinson, J.L.; Lee, M. *A Brief History of Physical Education*; Ronald Press: New York, NY, USA, 1969.
10. Kurz, D. Von der vielfalt sportlichen sinns zu den pädagogischen perspektiven im schulsport. In *Sportpädagogik: Ein Arbeitstextbuch*; Kuhlmann, D., Balz, E., Eds.; Federal Institute of Sport Science: Hamburg, Germany, 2008; pp. 162–173.
11. Lloyd, M.; Colley, R.C.; Tremblay, M.S. Advancing the debate on 'fitness testing' for children: Perhaps we're riding the wrong animal. *Pediatr. Exerc. Sci.* **2010**, *22*, 176–182. [CrossRef] [PubMed]
12. United Nations Educational Scientific and Cultural Organization (UNESCO). *Quality Physical Education*; United Nations Educational Scientific and Cultural Organization (UNESCO): Paris, France, 2015.
13. Whitehead, M. The concept of physical literacy. In *Physical Literacy: Throughout the Lifecourse*; Whitehead, M., Ed.; Routledge: London, UK, 2010; pp. 10–20.

14. Tomporowski, P.D.; Lambourne, K.; Okumura, M.S. Physical activity interventions and childre's mental function: An introduction and overview. *Prev. Med.* **2011**, *52*, 3–9. [CrossRef] [PubMed]

15. Trudeau, F.; Shephard, R.J. Relationships of physical activity to brain health and the academic performance of schoolchildren. *Am. J. Lifestyle Med.* **2008**, *5*, 10. [CrossRef]

16. Demetriou, Y.; Höner, O. Physical activity interventions in the school setting: A systematic review. *Psychol. Sport Exerc.* **2012**, *13*, 186–196. [CrossRef]

17. Tittlbach, S.A.; Sygusch, R.; Brehm, W.; Woll, A.; Lampert, T.; Abele, A.E.; Bös, K. Association between physical activity and health in german adolescents. *Eur. J. Sport Sci.* **2011**, *11*, 283–291. [CrossRef]

18. Bös, K. *Deutscher Motorik-Test 6-18 (DMT 6-18) [German Motor Performance Text 6-18];* Federal Institute of Sport Science: Hamburg, Germany, 2009; p. S115.

19. Herrmann, C.; Seelig, H. *MOBAK-1: Motorische Basiskompetenzen in der 1. Klasse: Testmanual [MOBAK-1: Motor Basic Skills in First Grade: Testmanual];* Exercise and Health (DSBG) of the University of Basel: Basel, Switzerland, 2014.

20. Herrmann, C.; Seelig, H. *MOBAK-3: Motorische Basiskompetenzen in der 3. Klasse: Testmanual [MOBAK-3: Basic Motor Competencies in Third Grade. Testmanual];* Exercise and Health (DSBG) of the University of Basel: Basel, Switzerland, 2015.

21. Prochaska, J.J.; Sallis, J.F.; Long, B. A physical activity screening measure for use with adolescents in primary care. *Arch. Pediatr. Adolesc. Med.* **2001**, *155*, 554–559. [CrossRef] [PubMed]

22. Jekauc, D.; Wagner, M.O.; Kahlert, D.; Woll, A. Reliabilität und validität des momo-aktivitätsfragebogens für jugendliche (momo-afb). *Diagnostica* **2013**, *59*, 100–111. [CrossRef]

23. Markland, D.; Hardy, L. On the factorial and construct validity of the intrinsic motivation inventory: Conceptual and operational concerns. *Res. Q. Exerc. Sport* **1997**, *68*, 20–32. [CrossRef] [PubMed]

24. Mrazek, J.; Schuessler, P.; Brauer, H. ESU—Eine einstellungsskala zum sportunterricht [an attitude skale for physical education]. *Sportunterricht* **1982**, *31*, 93–97.

25. Demetriou, Y. *Health Promotion in Physical Education. Development and Evaluation of the Eight Week PE Programme "HealthyPEP" for Sixth Grade Students in Germany;* Schriften der Deutschen Vereinigung für Sportwissenschaft: Hamburg, Germany, 2013; Volume 229, p. 206 Bl.

26. Davidson, M.C.; Amso, D.; Anderson, L.C.; Diamond, A. Development of cognitive control and executive functions from 4 to 13 years: Evidence from manipulations of memory, inhibition, and task switching. *Neuropsychologia* **2006**, *44*, 2037–2078. [CrossRef] [PubMed]

27. Mullane, J.C.; Corkum, P.V.; Klein, R.M.; McLaughlin, E. Interference control in children with and without ADHD: A systematic review of flanker and simon task performance. *Child Neuropsychol.* **2009**, *15*, 321–342. [CrossRef] [PubMed]

28. Townsend, J.T.; Ashby, F.G. *Stochastic Modeling of Elementary Psychological Processes;* Cambridge University Press: Cambridge, UK, 1983.

29. Fu, Y.; Gao, Z.; Hannon, J.C.; Burns, R.D.; Brusseau, T.A. Effect of the spark program on physical activity, cardiorespiratory endurance, and motivation in middle-school students. *J. Phys. Act. Health* **2016**, *13*, 534–542. [CrossRef] [PubMed]

30. Burns, R.D.; Fu, Y.; Podlog, L.W. School-based physical activity interventions and physical activity enjoyment: A meta-analysis. *Prev. Med.* **2017**, *103*, 84–90. [CrossRef] [PubMed]

31. Haug, E.; Torsheim, T.; Sallis, J.F.; Samdal, O. The characteristics of the outdoor school environment associated with physical activity. *Health Educ. Res.* **2010**, *25*, 248–256. [CrossRef] [PubMed]

32. Ishii, K.; Shibata, A.; Sato, M.; Oka, K. Recess Physical activity and perceived school environment among elementary school children. *Int. J. Environ. Res. Public Health* **2014**, *11*, 7195–7206. [CrossRef] [PubMed]

33. Baggett, C.D.; Stevens, J.; Catellier, D.J.; Evenson, K.R.; McMurray, R.G.; He, K.; Treuth, M.S. Compensation or displacement of physical activity in middle-school girls: The trial of activity for adolescent girls. *Int. J. Obes.* **2010**, *34*, 1193–1199. [CrossRef] [PubMed]

34. Gomersall, S.R.; Rowlands, A.V.; English, C.; Maher, C.; Olds, T.S. The activitystat hypothesis the concept, the evidence and the methodologies. *Sports Med.* **2013**, *43*, 135–149. [CrossRef] [PubMed]

35. Bugge, A.; Moller, S.; Tarp, J.; Hillman, C.H.; Lima, R.A.; Gejl, A.K.; Klakk, H.; Wedderkopp, N. Influence of a 2-to 6-year physical education intervention on scholastic performance: The champs study-dk. *Scand. J. Med. Sci. Sports* **2018**, *28*, 228–236. [CrossRef] [PubMed]

36. Tarp, J.; Domazet, S.L.; Froberg, K.; Hillman, C.H.; Andersen, L.B.; Bugge, A. Effectiveness of a school-based physical activity intervention on cognitive performance in danish adolescents: Lcomotion-learning, cognition and motion—A cluster randomized controlled trial. *PLoS ONE* **2016**, *11*, 0158087. [CrossRef] [PubMed]

37. Sallis, J.F.; McKenzie, T.L.; Kolody, B.; Lewis, M.; Marshall, S.; Rosengard, P. Effects of health-related physical education on academic achievement: Project spark. *Res. Q. Exerc. Sport* **1999**, *70*, 127–134. [CrossRef] [PubMed]

38. Alvarez-Bueno, C.; Pesce, C.; Cavero-Redondo, I.; Sanchez-Lopez, M.; Martinez-Hortelano, J.A.; Martinez-Vizcaino, V. The effect of physical activity interventions on children's cognition and metacognition: A systematic review and meta-analysis. *J. Am. Acad. Child Adolesc. Psychiatry* **2017**, *56*, 729–738. [CrossRef] [PubMed]

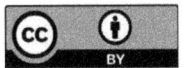

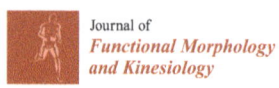

Journal of
*Functional Morphology
and Kinesiology*

Article

Actual vs. Perceived Motor Competence in Children (8–10 Years): An Issue of Non-Veridicality

Cain C. T. Clark [1,2,3,*], Jason Moran [1,2], Benjamin Drury [1,2], Fotini Venetsanou [4] and John F. T. Fernandes [1,2]

[1] Higher Education Sport, University Centre Hartpury, Gloucester GL19 3BE, UK;
jason.moran@hartpury.ac.uk (J.M.); ben.drury@hartpury.ac.uk (B.D.);
John.Fernandes@hartpury.ac.uk (J.F.T.F.)

[2] Sport, Exercise and Well-Being Research Arena, University Centre Hartpury, Gloucester GL19 3BE, UK

[3] Engineering Behaviour Analytics in Sports and Exercise (E-BASE) Research Group, Swansea University, Wales SA1 8EN, UK

[4] School of Physical Education and Sport Science National, Kapodistrian University of Athens, 17237 Athens, Greece; fvenetsanou@phed.uoa.gr

* Correspondence: cain.clark@hartpury.ac.uk; Tel.: +44-(0)-1452-702193

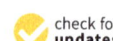

check for
updates

Received: 14 February 2018; Accepted: 20 March 2018; Published: 22 March 2018

Abstract: The purpose of this study was to investigate the between- and within-sex differences in actual and perceived locomotor and object control skills in children (8–10 year). All participants (58 children (29 boys; 9.5 ± 0.6 years; 1.44 ± 0.09 m; 39.6 ± 9.5 kg; body mass index; 18.8 ± 3.1 kg·m^2)) completed the Test of Gross Motor Development (2nd edition) and the Pictorial Scale of Perceived Movement Skill Competence for Young Children. Between- and within-sex differences were assessed using independent and paired samples t-tests, respectively. For all tests, effect sizes and Bayes factors were calculated. There were significant differences ($p < 0.001$) between sexes for perceived locomotor and perceived object control skills (boys > girls), with Bayes factors extremely in favour of the alternate hypothesis ($_{BF}$: 55,344 and 460, respectively). A significant difference ($p < 0.001$) was found between girls' actual and perceived locomotor skills ($d = -0.88$; 95% confidence interval: −0.46 to −1.34), with Bayes factors extremely in favour of the alternate hypothesis ($_{BF}$: 483). A significant difference ($p < 0.001$) was found between boys' actual and perceived object control skills ($d = 0.69$; 95% CI: 0.2 to 1.12), with Bayes factors very strongly in favour of the alternate hypothesis ($_{BF}$: 41). These findings suggest that there exists an issue of non-veridicality between actual and perceived motor competence skills, and their subsets, and a sex-mediated discord in children (8–10 years).

Keywords: motor competence; actual; perceived; children; locomotor; object control

---

1. Introduction

A substantial literature base now affirms the association between children's motor competence (MC) and physical activity (PA) behaviours, potentially, to combat the global obesity epidemic [1–4]. Motor competence refers to a child's ability to perform a wide range of motor skills in a proficient manner [5]. During early childhood, motor competence is frequently defined as proficiency in the performance of fundamental motor skills (FMS) [3,6]. Fundamental motor skills are considered to be the basic building blocks to more advanced movement patterns [7], and generally consist of locomotor and object control skills. Locomotor skills necessitate moving the body from one position to another (i.e., running, leaping, jumping, and galloping) while object control skills either refer to the receiving or propulsion of an object with the hand or foot (i.e., throwing, kicking, striking, and catching) [8].

Despite the mounting evidence for the benefit of qualifying contextual MC or movement quality data, there remains an over-predominance in focusing on the quantity of activity, rather than the quality [9,10]. Only recently has there been a trend towards a joint consideration of exercise quantity and quality [9–14]. A pivotal meta-analysis highlighted that PA interventions dedicated to improving quantity of PA report little effect [15]. More recently, Adab et al. [16] reported in a longitudinal study that a one-year school/community-based PA intervention had no effect on body mass index (BMI) z-scores at 15- or 30-months post-intervention, highlighting that communities and schools are unlikely to impact on the childhood obesity epidemic by incorporating only PA targeted interventions.

Given the above evidence, it is clear that the approach to PA promotion in youths must move beyond the mere use of caloric expenditure as the primary measure of exercise intensity. This notion has been largely influenced by the agglomerative evidence on the complex and dynamic interrelationships between weight status, health-related fitness, and motor and cognitive development through childhood and beyond [3,17–20]. Further, motor skill competence (i.e., the qualitative proficiency in performing an array of skills requiring motor coordination and control) has been highlighted for its positive associations with PA levels and health benefits in children and adolescents [21].

Stodden et al. [6] developed a comprehensive conceptual model that asserts that childhood MC is a determinant of health. Concomitantly, Barnett et al. [22] demonstrated, albeit prospectively, that childhood MC has a fundamental role for long-term PA compliance and is predictive of health-related fitness later in life. These pivotal works have prompted a new line of developmental research that, by means of cross-sectional, longitudinal, and experimental evidence [23], have confirmed the inveterate nature of the Stodden et al. [6] conceptual model. Interestingly, children's perception of being competent, and not MC per se, matters for promoting and adhering to an active lifestyle, which is necessary for positive trajectories of health and well-being [24]. Longitudinal research has identified perceived MC as a mechanism through which motor skill proficiency in childhood contributes to a physically active and healthy lifestyle in adolescence [25–28]. Given the influence that both actual and perceived MC in childhood can have as health determinants, empirical research has focused on furthering our understanding of their dynamic and changing relationship throughout childhood and adolescence [6,29].

Masci et al. [30] highlight that children and adolescents with different MC-based profiles also differ in motivation to practice PA, and actual PA levels. Furthermore, perceived, more than actual competence, appears to determine motivation for PA participation in children [31]. In the studies of Bardid et al. [31] and De Meester et al. [32], primary school children with a higher perception of MC resulted in higher motivation with this motivation remaining even when a low level of actual motor proficiency was combined with high self-perception (i.e., overestimation). Commonality exists between the aforementioned studies in the form of (non) veridicality of the physical self-concept, defined as the relation between the subjective perception and the corresponding external validity criterion. However, this issue remains relatively unexplored [33].

A general axiom is that boys tend to be more physically active than their female counterparts [34,35], and generally display better object control skills than girls, however, evidence on sex differences in locomotor skills is equivocal [36,37]. Contentiously, many studies show that girls outperform boys in locomotor skills [26,38,39], whilst a comparable number of studies assert that boys have equal [40,41] or higher locomotor skill competence [42]. Concerning the perception of MC, sex differences seem to proliferate during child development [29,43,44]. Whilst some studies report that boys and girls around the pre-school years display equal perceptions of competence, from primary school years onward, higher self-perceptions in boys are consistently found [29,45–47]. Notwithstanding, differences between actual and perceived MC in young children are widespread, yet equivocal; as is the discord between sexes, which remains contentious and relatively unexplored. Therefore, the purpose of this study was to investigate the between- and within-sex differences in actual and perceived locomotor and object control skills in children (8–10 years).

2. Materials and Methods

2.1. Participants and Settings

A sample of 58 children (29 boys) (mean ± standard deviation: 9.5 ± 0.6 years, 1.44 ± 0.09 m, 39.6 ± 9.5 kg, body mass index: 18.8 ± 3.1 kg·m^2) from a primary school in the United Kingdom volunteered to take part in this study. Optimal sample size was calculated based upon the ability to detect a smallest unit change (raw score) of 0.5% and a generous between subject standard deviation of 2.0 (α = 0.05, power 0.95). This subsequently yielded a sample-size estimation of 57. To equalize the ratio of males to females, 58 participants were recruited and divided into two groups (29 males, 29 females). Prior to the research commencing, parental or legal guardian informed consent and child assent was attained. The study was conducted in agreement with the guidelines and policies of the institutional ethics committee, and in accordance with the Declaration of Helsinki (ETHICS201617, 14 December 2016).

2.2. Instruments and Procedures

Actual motor competence. Children's actual MC was measured using the Test of Gross Motor Development (2nd edition) (TGMD-2) [48]. The TGMD-2 includes 12 fundamental movement skills (six locomotor skills and six object control skills) and takes approximately 20 min to administer. The locomotor subtest consists of running, galloping, hopping, leaping, horizontal jumping, and sliding. The object control subtest contains striking a stationary ball, a stationary dribble, catching, kicking, overhand throwing, and underhand rolling. Following a visual demonstration, participants were asked to perform each skill twice. The TGMD-2 is a qualitative measure in which each skill is scored against performance criteria prescribed in an accompanying manual (three to five criteria per skill); the criteria were scored 1 (present) or 0 (absent). Ratings in each item were summed to compute scores for locomotor and object control skills (each score ranging from 0 to 48). The psychometric properties of the TGMD-2 have been evaluated and the manual reports excellent test-retest reliability and inter-rater reliability (r > 0.85) as well as a good internal consistency (Cronbach's α = 0.85 and 0.88 for locomotor and object control subtests, respectively). Construct, content, and concurrent validity have also been determined for children aged 3 to 10 years [48–50]. Two experienced assessors scored the TGMD-2, with excellent inter-rater reliability (ICC: 0.99).

Perceived Motor Competence. Children's perceived MC was assessed via The Pictorial Scale of Perceived Movement Skill Competence for Young Children (PSPMSC) [51] for the same locomotor and object control skills as the TGMD-2. The perceived MC assessment took approximately 10 min to administer. For each skill, children were shown two sex-specific illustrations of a child performing the skill in competent and less-competent ways. Children were asked which depiction they identified themselves with the most, with each question having the same standard structure: "This child is pretty good at X, this child is not that good at X: Which child is most like you?". Once children selected a picture, they were then asked to further indicate their perceived MC as more or less identifying with the selected picture. For the picture of the most competent child, the follow-up question was: "Are you pretty good or really good at X?", for the picture of the less competent child, the accompanying question was: "Are you sort of good or not that good at X?"; each item was scored 1 (not that good), 2 (sort of good), 3 (pretty good), or 4 (really good). Scores for locomotor and object control skills were summed to compute scores for locomotor and object control skills (each score ranging from 6 to 24). The PSPMSC has been shown to have acceptable face validity as well good test-retest reliability (r > 0.78) and internal consistency (Cronbach's α = 0.60–0.81; Barnett et al. [51]). Construct validity has also been established in children aged 4 to 10 years [48–50,52].

2.3. Data Analysis

Raw scores for the TGMD-2 and The PSPMSC were transformed into percentiles to facilitate statistical analyses, per manual guidelines [48]. Data were initially assessed for normality using a Shapiro-Wilk test, and found to be normally distributed ($p > 0.05$). Subsequently, between-sex differences for actual locomotor, actual object control, perceived locomotor, and perceived object control percentiles were assessed using independent samples t-tests. Within-sex differences for actual vs. perceived locomotor and object control percentiles were assessed using paired samples t-tests. Bayesian statistical analyses were conducted for within- and between-sex differences utilizing default priors [53–55], where Bayes factors expressing the probability of the data given H_{10} (alternate hypothesis) relative to H_{01} (null hypothesis; i.e., values larger than 1 are in favour of H_1) assuming that H_{01} and H_{10} are equally likely, were produced. Data were reported as mean $\pm$ SD, with effect sizes (Cohen's d, classified as: small (0.2), medium (0.5), large (0.8), or very large (1.3) [56] and 95% confidence intervals (CIs)). The alpha level was set at 0.05 a priori. Bayes factors were reported as the probability of the data given the alternate, relative to the null hypothesis, or vice-versa (classified as: anecdotal ($_{BF}$1–3), moderate ($_{BF}$3–10), strong ($_{BF}$10–30), very strong ($_{BF}$30–100), or extreme ($_{BF} > 100$)) [53–55]. All data analyses were conducted using the JASP statistical package (JASP Team, 2018, jasp-stats.org; version 0.8.6, University of Amsterdam, Amsterdam, The Netherlands).

3. Results

3.1. Between-Sex Differences

There was no significant difference ($p = 0.15$) found between sexes for actual locomotor skills (Female (F): 69.8 $\pm$ 5.27 vs. Male (M): 72.3 $\pm$ 7.47%; $d = 0.38$, 95% CI: 0.14 to 0.9) (Figure 1). Bayes factors found anecdotal evidence in favour of the null vs. alternate hypothesis ($_{BF}$: 1.5, i.e., null 1.5 times more probable than the alternate).

There was no significant difference ($p = 0.87$) found between sexes for actual object control skills (F: 62.75 $\pm$ 10.5 vs. M: 63.3 $\pm$ 15.2%; $d = 0.04$, 95% CI: -0.56 to 0.47) (Figure 1). Bayes factors found moderate evidence in favour of the null vs. alternate hypothesis ($_{BF}$: 3.72, i.e., null 3.72 times more probable than the alternate).

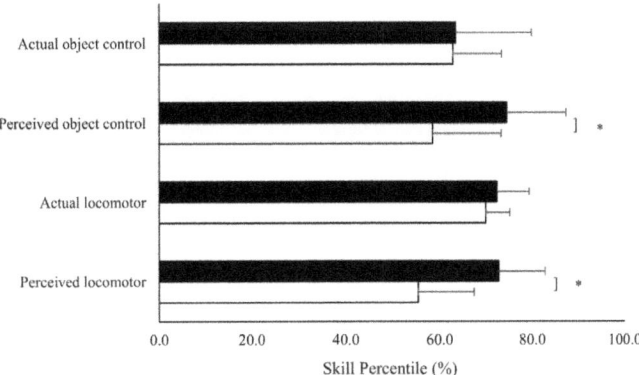

Figure 1. Between-sex perceived and actual locomotor and object control skill percentile scores. Black bars denote boys; white bars denote girls; * denotes significant difference between sexes ($p < 0.05$).

There was a significant difference ($p < 0.001$) found between sexes for perceived locomotor skills (F: 55.46 $\pm$ 11.8 vs. M: 72.7 $\pm$ 10.2%; $d = 1.6$, 95% CI: 0.95 to 2.14) (Figure 1). Bayes factors found extreme evidence in favour of the alternative vs. null hypothesis ($_{BF}$: 55,344, i.e., alternate 55,244 times more probable than the null).

There was a significant difference ($p < 0.001$) found between sexes for perceived object control skills (F: 58.5 $\pm$ 14.7 vs. M: 74.4 $\pm$ 12.6%; $d = 1.17$, 95% CI: 0.6 to 1.71) (Figure 1). Bayes factors found extreme evidence in favour of the alternate vs. null hypothesis ($_{BF}$: 460, i.e., alternate 460 times more probable than the null).

3.2. Within-Sex Differences

There was a significant difference ($p < 0.001$) found between girls' actual and perceived locomotor skills (Actual 69.8 ± 5.2 vs. Perceived 55.5 ± 11.9%; $d = -0.88$, 95% CI: −0.46 to −1.34) (Figure 2). Bayes factors found extreme evidence in favour of the alternative vs. null hypothesis ($_{BF}$: 483, i.e., alternate 483 times more probable than the null).

There was no significant difference ($p = 0.06$) found between girls' actual and perceived object control skills (Actual 62.8 ± 10.5 vs. Perceived 58.4 ± 14.7%; $d = -0.36$, 95% CI: −0.02 to −0.74) (Figure 2). Bayes factors found anecdotal evidence in favour of the null vs. alternate hypothesis ($_{BF}$: 1.01, i.e., null 1.01 times more probable than the alternate).

There was no significant difference ($p = 0.84$) found between boys' actual and perceived locomotor skills (Actual 72.3 ± 7.5 vs. Perceived 72.7 ± 10.2%; $d = 0.04$, 95% CI: −0.41 to 0.33) (Figure 2). Bayes factors found moderate evidence in favour of the null vs. alternate hypothesis ($_{BF}$: 4.97, i.e., null 4.97 times more probable than the alternate).

There was a significant difference ($p < 0.001$) between boys' actual and perceived object control skills (Actual 63.3 ± 16.2 vs. Perceived 74.4 ± 10.2%; $d = 0.69$, 95% CI: 0.2 to 1.12) (Figure 2). Bayes factors found very strong evidence in favour of the alternative vs. null hypothesis ($_{BF}$: 41, i.e., alternate 41 times more probable than the null).

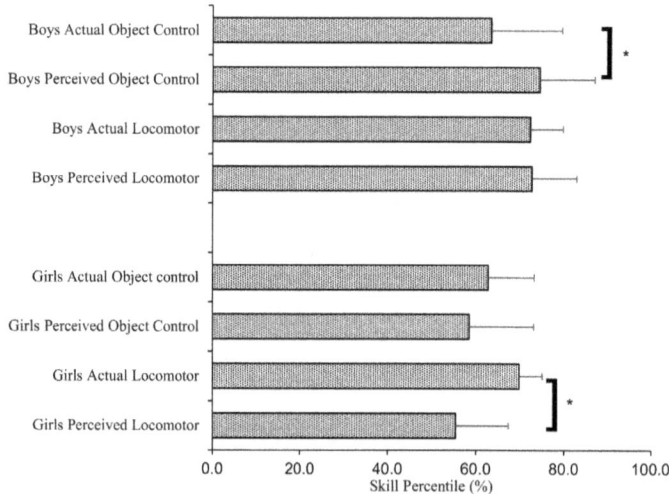

Figure 2. Within-sex differences for perceived and actual locomotor and object control skill percentile scores. * denotes significant difference between actual and perceived scores ($p < 0.05$).

4. Discussion

The purpose of this study was to investigate the between- and within-sex differences in actual and perceived locomotor and object control skills in children (8–10 years). In accord with the aforementioned purpose, the key findings of this study were:

(1)   Boys perceived their locomotor and object control skills to be greater than girls.
(2)   Girls perceived their locomotor skills to be lower than their actual locomotor skills.
(3)   Boys perceived their object control skills to be greater than their actual object control skills.

4.1. Between-Sex Differences

Evidence on sex differences in locomotor skills is equivocal [26,36,37,57]. Contentiously, many studies show that girls outperform boys in their locomotor skills [26,38,39], whilst almost an equal number of studies assert that boys have equal [40,41] or higher locomotor skill competence [42]. It is, therefore, unsurprising that the findings of the present study should be equally equivocal for actual MC (locomotor and object control). There was no significant difference ($p = 0.15$) between boys and girls for actual locomotor skills (Figure 1), highlighting very little discord in actual locomotor skills between sexes. Furthermore, Bayes factors indicated that there was only anecdotal evidence to separate the null and alternate hypotheses. Similarly, there was no significant difference ($p = 0.87$) between sexes for actual object control skills (Figure 1), further supporting the observations of Bardid et al. [31] and Slykerman et al. [41].

There was a significant difference ($p < 0.001$) found between sexes for perceived locomotor skills, where boys perceived themselves to be ~20 percentage points higher than girls (Figure 1). This is supported by Bayes factors analysis, which found extreme evidence in favour of the alternative vs. null hypothesis ($_{\text{BF}}$: 55,344). Similarly, boys also perceived their object control skills to be greater than that of the girls, with a significant difference ($p < 0.001$) found between sexes (Figure 1). Bayes factors found 'extreme' evidence in favour of there being a difference between sexes ($_{\text{BF}}$: 460). Whilst the present study highlights differences in perceived, but not in actual, object control and locomotor skills, Brian et al. [58] concluded that there was relatively little sex-related discord for perceived and actual locomotor skills, however, there were evident differences for perceived and actual object control skills. This difference is likely influenced by age, with Brian et al. [58] assessing 4- to 5-year-olds, contrasting with the 8- to 10-year-olds in the present study. Concerning the perception of MC, sex-mediated differences are found to proliferate during child development [43,44]. The modal finding in the literature is that boys and girls around the pre-school years display equal perceptions of competence [59,60]. However, from primary school years onward, higher self-perceptions in boys are consistently found [45,46], which supports the findings in the present study.

4.2. Non-Veridicality in Boys and Girls

Masci et al. [30] highlighted low agreement between motor skill competence perceived by children and their actual skill observed by experts, as the percentage of variance of perceived competence explained by actual competence was low (5% and 6% for locomotor and object control skills, respectively). The authors speculated that this was due to the low accuracy of self-perceptions when cognitive capabilities necessary to make a realistic domain-specific self-evaluation are still immature [43,44]. Substantial evidence suggests that girls have lower perceived and actual ball skill competence than boys as early as young childhood [26,38,39,51,61]. Independently of their actual proficiency level, Masci et al. [30] suggest that girls more frequently underestimated their actual object control skills than boys. The observation that girls more frequently underestimate their actual object control skills compared to boys may be pertinent in light of evidence that object control skills predict involvement in PA and health-related fitness later in life [25,57,62]. Further, evidence suggests that the perception of competence in object control skills mediates the translation of actual MC into health-related outcomes [22,51,62]. The present study supports these findings, but for boys only, where a significant difference ($p < 0.001$) was found between boys' actual and perceived object control skills (Figure 2). Further, Bayes factors confirmed, very strongly, in favour of the alternative vs. null hypothesis ($_{\text{BF}}$: 41). Whilst, conversely, for girls, with regards to object control skills, high veridicality was displayed, with only a small, negative effect size being found (Figure 2).

Masci et al. [30] reported that around one quarter of boys overestimated their object and locomotor control skills more frequently than girls. The present study supports the inference that boys overestimate and girls underestimate MC levels. Interestingly, this study also found that actual levels of locomotor and object control skills were comparable between boys and girls. Despite this, a large sex-mediated discord was evident for girls' locomotor skills, indicating that they systematically under-perceived their actual locomotor competence. Boys, however, systematically over-perceived their actual object control skills. De Meester et al. [63] noted four distinct groups for actual and perceived MC: two groups with high veridicality, i.e., high actual and high perceived, or low actual and low perceived MC. However, the authors also identified a subset of their sample that systematically over- or underestimated its actual MC skill. Interestingly, the strongest correlate of high PA and low BMI was not high actual MC, but high perceived MC. Furthermore, in a comparable population, De Meester et al. [63] found no apparent sex-mediated discord, yet De Meester et al. [32] highlighted this as an issue. Whilst the present study focused on the sex-mediated differences between actual and perceived MC, and not the concept of over- or under-estimation, the present findings are in general concordance with recent evidence [30,63].

4.3. Limitations

One limitation of the present study is its cross-sectional design. Causal inference cannot be assumed regarding actual MC and perceived MC. To gain more insight into these differences and to understand how differences within- and between-the sexes may change or develop over time, longitudinal studies must be conducted. Another possible limitation is the use of a convenience sample, which may result in under- or over-representation of particular groups within a sample but should not detract from the suitably (statistically) powered nature of the study.

5. Conclusions

To the authors' knowledge, this is the first study to assess between- and within-sex differences for actual and perceived locomotor and object control skills. Furthermore, this would appear to be the first study to incorporate Bayes factor inferences in the analyses of children's MC.

The finding that boys' and girls' actual locomotor and actual object control skills are comparable, despite differences in perceptions, is in line with current literature. The novel analytical approach taken in this study to focus on sex-mediated differences in MC adds clarity to an equivocal set of results in the literature. Given the large (effect sizes) and extreme (Bayes factors) differences found between actual and perceived locomotor and object control skills, it is clear that non-veridicality, with regard to MC, in young children is a problem. Further, the propensity of young boys and girls to over or under perceive their PA-related skills, respectively, needs to be acknowledged and addressed by, in particular, schools and key stakeholders in children's PA, and this should be considered in any related intervention. It is advisable that future research considers not only variable and person-centred approaches, but also the clear sex-mediated differences in perceived and actual MC, including its subsets, and the impact on PA.

Acknowledgments: The authors wish to acknowledge the time, effort, and dedication of the children involved in this study.

Author Contributions: Cain C. T. Clark conceived and designed the experiments; Cain C. T. Clark performed the experiments; Cain C. T. Clark and John F. T. Fernandes analysed the data; Cain C. T. Clark, Benjamin Drury, Fotini Venetsanou, John F. T. Fernandes, and Jason Moran wrote the paper.

Conflicts of Interest: The authors declare no conflict of interest.

References

1. Figueroa, R.; An, R. Motor skill competence and physical activity in preschoolers: A review. *Matern. Child Health J.* **2017**, *21*, 136–146. [CrossRef] [PubMed]
2. Holfelder, B.; Schott, N. Relationship of fundamental movement skills and physical activity in children and adolescents: A systematic review. *Psychol. Sport Exerc.* **2014**, *15*, 382–391. [CrossRef]
3. Logan, S.W.; Webster, K.; Getchell, N.; Pfeiffer, K.; Robinson, L.E. Relationship between fundamental motor skill competence and physical activity during childhood and adolescence: A systematic review. *Kines. Rev.* **2015**, *4*, 416–426. [CrossRef]
4. Clark, C.C.T. Is obesity *actually* non-communicable? *Obes. Med.* **2017**, *8*, 27–28. [CrossRef]

5. Haga, M. The relationship between physical fitness and motor competence in children. *Child. Care Health Dev.* **2008**, *34*, 329–334. [CrossRef] [PubMed]

6. Stodden, D.F.; Goodway, J.D.; Langendorfer, S.J.; Roberton, M.A.; Rudisill, M.E.; Garcia, C.; Garcia, L.E. A developmental perspective on the role of motor skill competence in physical activity: An emergent relationship. *Quest* **2008**, *60*, 290–306. [CrossRef]

7. Seefeldt, V. Developmental motor patterns: Implications for elementary school physical education. In *Psychology of Motor Behaviour and Sport*; Nadeau, C., Holliwell, W., Newell, K., Roberts, G., Eds.; Human Kinetics: Champaign, IL, USA, 1980; pp. 314–323.

8. Gallahue, D.L.; Ozmun, J.C.; Goodway, J.D. *Understanding Motor Development: Infants, Children, Adolescents, Adults*, 7th ed.; McGraw Hill: Boston, MA, USA, 2011.

9. Clark, C.C.T. Profiling movement and gait quality using accelerometry in children's physical activity: Consider quality, not just quantity. *Br. J. Sports Med.* **2017**. [CrossRef] [PubMed]

10. Clark, C.C.T.; Barnes, C.M.; Swindell, N.J.; Holton, M.D.; Bingham, D.D.; Collings, P.J.; Barber, S.E.; Summers, H.D.; Mackintosh, K.A.; Stratton, G. Profiling movement and gait quality characteristics in pre-school children. *J. Motor Behav.* **2017**, 1–9. [CrossRef] [PubMed]

11. Barnes, C.M.; Clark, C.C.; Holton, M.D.; Stratton, G.; Summers, H.D. Quantitative time profiling of children's activity and motion. *Med. Sci. Sports Exerc.* **2017**, *49*, 183–190. [CrossRef] [PubMed]

12. Clark, C.C.T.; Barnes, C.M.; Holton, M.D.; Summers, H.D.; Stratton, G. Profiling movement quality and gait characteristics according to body-mass index in children (9–11 y). *Hum. Mov. Sci.* **2016**, *49*, 291–300. [CrossRef] [PubMed]

13. Clark, C.C.T.; Barnes, C.M.; Summers, H.D.; Mackintosh, K.A.; Stratton, G. Profiling movement quality characteristics of children (9–11 y) during recess. *Eur. J. Hum. Mov.* **2018**, *39*, 143–160.

14. Garber, C.E.; Blissmer, B.; Deschenes, M.R.; Franklin, B.A.; Lamonte, M.J.; Lee, I.M.; Nieman, D.C.; Swain, D.P.; American College of Sports; American college of sports medicine position stand. Quantity and quality of exercise for developing and maintaining cardiorespiratory, musculoskeletal, and neuromotor fitness in apparently healthy adults: Guidance for prescribing exercise. *Med. Sci. Sports Exerc.* **2011**, *43*, 1334–1359. [PubMed]

15. Metcalf, B.; Henley, W.; Wilkin, T. Republished research: Effectiveness of intervention on physical activity of children: Systematic review and meta-analysis of controlled trials with objectively measured outcomes (earlybird 54). *Br. J. Sports Med.* **2013**, *47*, 226. [CrossRef] [PubMed]

16. Adab, P.; Pallan, M.; Lancashire, E.R.; Hemming, K.; Frew, E.; Barrett, T.; Bhopal, R.; Cade, J.; Canaway, A.; Clarke, J.; et al. Effectiveness of a childhood obesity prevention programme delivered through schools, targeting 6 and 7 years olds: Cluster randomised controlled trial (waves study). *BMJ* **2018**, *360*, k211. [CrossRef] [PubMed]

17. D'Hondt, E.; Deforche, B.; Gentier, I.; Verstuyf, J.; Vaeyens, R.; De Bourdeaudhuij, I.; Philippaerts, R.; Lenoir, M. A longitudinal study of gross motor coordination and weight status in children. *Obesity* **2014**, *22*, 1505–1511. [CrossRef] [PubMed]

18. Reinert, K.R.; Poe, E.K.; Barkin, S.L. The relationship between executive function and obesity in children and adolescents: A systematic literature review. *J. Obes.* **2013**, *2013*, 820956. [CrossRef] [PubMed]

19. Rodrigues, L.P.; Stodden, D.F.; Lopes, V.P. Developmental pathways of change in fitness and motor competence are related to overweight and obesity status at the end of primary school. *J. Sci. Med. Sport Sports Med. Aust.* **2016**, *19*, 87–92. [CrossRef] [PubMed]

20. Lopes, V.P.; Stodden, D.F.; Rodrigues, L.P. Weight status is associated with cross-sectional trajectories of motor co-ordination across childhood. *Child Care Health Dev.* **2014**, *40*, 891–899. [CrossRef] [PubMed]

21. Lubans, D.R.; Morgan, P.J.; Cliff, D.P.; Barnett, L.M.; Okely, A.D. Fundamental movement skills in children and adolescents: Review of associated health benefits. *Sports Med.* **2010**, *40*, 1019–1035. [CrossRef] [PubMed]

22. Barnett, L.M.; Van Beurden, E.; Morgan, P.J.; Brooks, L.O.; Beard, J.R. Does childhood motor skill proficiency predict adolescent fitness? *Med. Sci. Sports Exerc.* **2008**, *40*, 2137–2144. [CrossRef] [PubMed]

23. Robinson, L.E.; Stodden, D.F.; Barnett, L.M.; Lopes, V.P.; Logan, S.W.; Rodrigues, L.P.; D'Hondt, E. Motor competence and its effect on positive developmental trajectories of health. *Sports Med.* **2015**, *45*, 1273–1284. [CrossRef] [PubMed]

24. Inchley, J.; Kirby, J.; Currie, C. Longitudinal changes in physical self-perceptions and associations with physical activity during adolescence. *Pediatr. Exerc. Sci.* **2011**, *23*, 237–249. [CrossRef] [PubMed]

25.	Barnett, L.M.; Morgan, P.J.; Van Beurden, E.; Ball, K.; Lubans, D.R. A reverse pathway? Actual and perceived skill proficiency and physical activity. *Med. Sci. Sports Exerc.* **2011**, *43*, 898–904. [CrossRef] [PubMed]

26.	Barnett, L.M.; Morgan, P.J.; van Beurden, E.; Beard, J.R. Perceived sports competence mediates the relationship between childhood motor skill proficiency and adolescent physical activity and fitness: A longitudinal assessment. *Int. J. Behav. Nutr. Phys. Act.* **2008**, *5*, 40. [CrossRef] [PubMed]

27.	Khodaverdi, Z.; Bahram, A.; Khalaji, H.; Kazemnejad, A. Motor skill competence and perceived motor competence: Which best predicts physical activity among girls? *Iran. J. Public Health* **2013**, *42*, 1145–1150. [PubMed]

28.	Khodaverdi, Z.; Bahram, A.; Robinson, L.E. Correlates of physical activity behaviours in young Iranian girls. *Child Care Health Dev.* **2015**, *41*, 903–910. [CrossRef] [PubMed]

29.	True, L.; Brian, A.; Goodway, J.; Stodden, D. Relationships between product- and process-oriented measures of motor competence and perceived competence. *J. Motor Learn. Dev.* **2017**, *5*, 319–335. [CrossRef]

30.	Masci, I.; Schmidt, M.; Marchetti, R.; Vannozzi, G.; Pesce, C. When children's perceived and actual motor competence mismatch: Sport participation and gender differences. *J. Motor Learn. Dev.* **2017**, *0*, 1–33. [CrossRef]

31.	Bardid, F.; de Meester, A.; Tallir, I.; Cardon, G.; Lenoir, M.; Haerens, L. Configurations of actual and perceived motor competence among children: Associations with motivation for sports and global self-worth. *Hum. Mov. Sci.* **2016**, *50*, 1–9. [CrossRef] [PubMed]

32.	De Meester, A.; Stodden, D.; Brian, A.; True, L.; Cardon, G.; Tallir, I.; Haerens, L. Associations among elementary school children's actual motor competence, perceived motor competence, physical activity and bmi: A cross-sectional study. *PLoS ONE* **2016**, *11*, e0164600. [CrossRef] [PubMed]

33.	Schmidt, M.; Valkanover, S.; Conzelmann, A. Veridicality of self-concept of strength in male adolescents. *Percept. Motor Skills* **2013**, *116*, 1029–1042. [CrossRef] [PubMed]

34.	Gortmaker, S.L.; Lee, R.; Cradock, A.L.; Sobol, A.M.; Duncan, D.T.; Wang, Y.C. Disparities in youth physical activity in the United States: 2003–2006. *Med. Sci. Sports Exerc.* **2012**, *44*, 888–893. [CrossRef] [PubMed]

35.	Schmutz, E.A.; Leeger-Aschmann, C.S.; Radtke, T.; Muff, S.; Kakebeeke, T.H.; Zysset, A.E.; Messerli-Burgy, N.; Stulb, K.; Arhab, A.; Meyer, A.H.; et al. Correlates of preschool children's objectively measured physical activity and sedentary behavior: A cross-sectional analysis of the splashy study. *Int. J. Behav. Nutr. Phys. Act.* **2017**, *14*, 1. [CrossRef] [PubMed]

36.	Barnett, L.; Stodden, D.F.; Cohen, K.E.; Smith, J.J.; Lubans, D.R.; Lenoir, M.; Iivonen, S.; Miller, A.; Laukkanen, A.; Dudley, D.A.; et al. Fundamental movement skills: An important focus. *J. Teach. Phys. Educ.* **2016**, *35*, 219–225. [CrossRef]

37.	Barnett, L.M.; Lai, S.K.; Veldman, S.L.C.; Hardy, L.L.; Cliff, D.P.; Morgan, P.J.; Zask, A.; Lubans, D.R.; Shultz, S.P.; Ridgers, N.D.; et al. Correlates of gross motor competence in children and adolescents: A systematic review and meta-analysis. *Sports Med.* **2016**, *46*, 1663–1688. [CrossRef] [PubMed]

38.	Hardy, L.L.; King, L.; Farrell, L.; Macniven, R.; Howlett, S. Fundamental movement skills among Australian preschool children. *J. Sci. Med. Sport* **2010**, *13*, 503–508. [CrossRef] [PubMed]

39.	Liong, G.H.; Ridgers, N.D.; Barnett, L.M. Associations between skill perceptions and young children's actual fundamental movement skills. *Percept. Motor Skills* **2015**, *120*, 591–603. [CrossRef] [PubMed]

40.	Bardid, F.; Huyben, F.; Lenoir, M.; Seghers, J.; Martelaer, K.; Goodway, J.; Deconinck, F.J. Asseessment fundamental motor skills in Belgian children aged 208 years highlights differences in us reference sample. *Acta Paediatr.* **2016**, *105*, e281–e290. [CrossRef] [PubMed]

41.	Slykerman, S.; Ridgers, N.D.; Stevenson, C.; Barnett, L.M. How important is young children's actual and perceived movement skill competence to their physical activity? *J. Sci. Med. Sport Sports Med. Aust.* **2016**, *19*, 488–492. [CrossRef] [PubMed]

42.	Robinson, L.E. The relationship between perceived physical competence and fundamental motor skills in preschool children. *Child. Care Health Dev.* **2011**, *37*, 589–596. [CrossRef] [PubMed]

43.	Harter, S. The development of self-presentations during childhood and adolescnece. In *Handbook of Self and Identity*; Leary, M.R., Tangney, J.P., Eds.; Wiley & Sons: New York, NY, USA, 2005.

44.	Harter, S. The self. In *Handbook of Child Psychology: Vol 3. Soical, Emotional and Persoanlity Development*; Damon, R., Lerner, M.R., Eds.; Wiley & Sons: New York, NY, USA, 2006.

45.	Fredricks, J.A.; Eccles, J. Children's competence and value beliefs from childhood through adolescence: Growth trajectories in two male-sex-typed domains. *Dev. Psychol.* **2002**, *38*, 519–533. [CrossRef] [PubMed]

46. Noordstar, J.J.; van der Net, J.; Jak, S.; Helders, P.J.; Jongmans, M.J. Global self-esteem, perceived athletic comptence, and physical activity in children: A longitudinal cohort study. *Psychol. Sport Exerc.* **2016**, *22*, 83–90. [CrossRef]

47. Jacobs, J.E.; Lanza, S.; Osgood, D.W.; Eccles, J.S.; Wigfield, A. Changes in children's self-competence and values: Gender and domain differences across grades one through twelve. *Child. Dev.* **2002**, *73*, 509–527. [CrossRef] [PubMed]

48. Ulrich, D.A. *Test. of Gross Motor Development: Examiner's Manual*, 2nd ed.; PRO-ED: Austin, TX, USA, 2000.

49. Kim, C.; Han, D.; Park, I. Reliability and validity of the test of gross motor development-2 in Korean preschool children. *Res. Dev. Dis.* **2014**, *2*, 2–9.

50. Valentini, N. Validity and reliability of the tgmd-2 for Brazilian children. *J. Motor Behav.* **2012**, *44*, 275–280. [CrossRef] [PubMed]

51. Barnett, L.M.; Ridgers, N.D.; Salmon, J. Associations between young children's perceived and actual ball skill competence and physical activity. *J. Sci. Med. Sport* **2015**, *18*, 167–171. [CrossRef] [PubMed]

52. Barnett, L.M.; Robinson, L.E.; Webster, E.K.; Ridgers, N.D. Reliability of the pictorial scale of perceived movement skill competence in 2 diverse samples of young children. *J. Phys. Act. Health* **2015**, *12*, 1045–1051. [CrossRef] [PubMed]

53. Wagenmakers, E.J.; Marsman, M.; Jamil, T.; Ly, A.; Verhagen, J.; Love, J.; Selker, R.; Gronau, Q.F.; Smira, M.; Epskamp, S.; et al. Bayesian inference for psychology. Part I: Theoretical advantages and practical ramifications. *Psychon. Bull. Rev.* **2017**, *25*, 35–57. [CrossRef] [PubMed]

54. Wagenmakers, E.J.; Love, J.; Marsman, M.; Jamil, T.; Ly, A.; Verhagen, J.; Selker, R.; Gronau, Q.F.; Dropmann, D.; Boutin, B.; et al. Bayesian inference for psychology. Part II: Example applications with JASP. *Psychon. Bull. Rev.* **2017**, *25*, 58–76. [CrossRef] [PubMed]

55. Marsman, M.; Wagenmakers, E.J. Bayesian benefits with jasp. *Eur. J. Dev. Psychol.* **2016**, *14*, 545–555. [CrossRef]

56. Cohen, J. *Statistical Power Analysis for the Behavioral Sciences*, 3rd ed.; Lawrence Erlbaum Associates: New York, NY, USA, 1988.

57. Barnett, L.M.; Ridgers, N.D.; Hesketh, K.; Salmon, J. Setting them up for lifetime activity: Play competence perceptions and physical activity in young children. *J. Sci. Med. Sport Sports Med. Aust.* **2017**, *20*, 856–860. [CrossRef] [PubMed]

58. Brian, A.; Bardid, F.; Barnett, L.; Deconinck, F.J.; Lenoir, M.; Goodway, J. Actual and perceived motor competence levels of Belgian and US preschool children. *J. Motor Learn. Dev.* **2017**, 1–29. [CrossRef]

59. Breslin, G.; Murphy, M.; McKee, D.; Delaney, B.; Dempster, M. The effect of teachers trained in a fundamental movement skills programme on children's slef-perceptions and motor competence. *Eur. Phys. Educ. Rev.* **2012**, *18*, 114–126. [CrossRef]

60. Crane, J.R.; Naylor, P.J.; Cook, R.; Temple, V.A. Do perceptions of competence mediate the relationship between fundamental motor skill proficiency and physical activity levels of children in kindergarten? *J. Phys. Act. Health* **2015**, *12*, 954–961. [CrossRef] [PubMed]

61. Barnett, L.M.; Ridgers, N.D.; Zask, A.; Salmon, J. Face validity and reliability of a pictorial instrument for assessing fundamental movement skill perceived competence in young children. *J. Sci. Med. Sport Sports Med. Aust.* **2015**, *18*, 98–102. [CrossRef] [PubMed]

62. Barnett, L.M.; van Beurden, E.; Morgan, P.J.; Brooks, L.O.; Beard, J.R. Childhood motor skill proficiency as a predictor of adolescent physical activity. *J. Adolesc. Health Off. Pub. Soc. Adolesc. Med.* **2009**, *44*, 252–259. [CrossRef] [PubMed]

63. De Meester, A.; Maes, J.; Stodden, D.; Cardon, G.; Goodway, J.; Lenoir, M.; Haerens, L. Identifying profiles of actual and perceived motor competence among adolescents: Associations with motivation, physical activity, and sports participation. *J. Sports Sci.* **2016**, *34*, 2027–2037. [CrossRef] [PubMed]

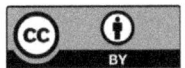

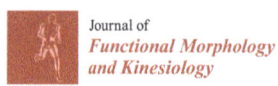

Journal of
Functional Morphology
and Kinesiology

Article

Relationship between Sedentary Time, Physical Activity and Multiple Lifestyle Factors in Children

Michael P. R. Sheldrick *, Richard Tyler, Kelly A. Mackintosh and Gareth Stratton

Research Centre in Applied Sports, Technology, Exercise and Medicine (A-STEM), Swansea University,
Swansea SA2 8PP, UK; 839039@swansea.ac.uk (R.T.); k.mackintosh@swansea.ac.uk (K.A.M.);
g.stratton@swansea.ac.uk (G.S.)
* Correspondence: 708824@swansea.ac.uk; Tel.: +44-7749-767373

Received: 12 December 2017; Accepted: 22 February 2018; Published: 2 March 2018

Abstract: An improved understanding of relationships between moderate-to-vigorous physical activity (MVPA), screen-time and lifestyle factors is imperative for developing interventions, yet few studies have explored such relationships simultaneously. Therefore, the study's aim was to examine the relationship between sufficient MVPA ($\geq$60 min·day^{-1}) and excessive screen-time ($\geq$2 h·day^{-1}) with lifestyle factors in children. In total, 756 children (10.4 ± 0.6 years) completed a questionnaire, which assessed sleep duration, MVPA, homework/reading, screen-time and diet, and a 20 metre multi-stage shuttle run test to assess cardiorespiratory fitness (CRF). Body mass and stature were measured and used to calculate BMI (body mass index) for age/sex z-scores. Fruit and vegetable consumption and CRF were positively associated with sufficient MVPA, irrespective of sex ($p < 0.05$). Excessive screen-time was positively associated with sugary snack consumption in boys and girls, and diet soft drink intake in boys ($p < 0.05$). In addition, excessive screen-time was negatively associated with MVPA before school for both boys and girls, as well as with sleep duration and fruit and vegetable consumption for girls ($p < 0.05$). Sufficient MVPA and excessive screen-time were associated with healthy and unhealthy factors, respectively, with relationships sometimes differing by sex. Future health promoting interventions should consider targeting change in multiple lifestyle factors.

Keywords: youth; moderate-to-vigorous physical activity; screen-time; health; diet; behaviours

1. Introduction

Childhood obesity is a major public health concern [1], particularly in Wales, which has the highest prevalence in the United Kingdom [2], and often tracks into adulthood [3]. Associated lifetime health risks are frequently cited, such as cardiovascular disease [4], type 2 diabetes [5] and other chronic diseases [6]. There is evidence that modifiable lifestyle factors, including physical inactivity [7], poor diet [8], insufficient sleep [9] and excessive sedentary behaviour [10] are key contributors to the obesity epidemic in children and all-cause mortality. Conversely, regular physical activity [7], adequate consumption of fruit and vegetables [11] and sufficient sleep [9] are widely accepted as protective. Of these lifestyle factors, physical activity and sedentary time have been identified as the most strongly associated with obesity and health [12,13].

As well as being shown to have a robust relationship with obesity, regular moderate-to-vigorous physical activity (MVPA) is also considered to be a preventative measure for poor cardiorespiratory fitness (CRF) and several other health risk factors in children [7]. The way by which MVPA improves health is not fully understood [7], but may be partially explained by its relationship with other healthy lifestyle factors [7,14,15]. Indeed, MVPA is associated with healthy dietary habits, such as increased fruit and vegetable consumption [15,16], breakfast consumption [17] and a lower intake of unhealthy sugary snacks [18]. Additionally, MVPA has been associated with improved cognitive function [19] and longer sleep duration [14], however relationships with the latter are equivocal [20,21]. Despite this, MVPA levels remain low among children of all ages with less than 20 percent meeting the current UK physical activity (PA) guidelines of at least 60 minutes MVPA every day [22]. Furthermore, even children meeting the PA guidelines [23] spend a large proportion of their discretionary time in sedentary behaviours (up to 9 h daily) [10].

Whilst homework and reading have been identified as prominent sedentary behaviours amongst children [24], screen-time remains the most prevalent [10] and has been consistently associated with obesity, poor CRF, cognitive function and overall cardio metabolic health [10]. Moreover, screen-time is associated with short sleep duration [25,26], less time spent in MVPA [15,27], a poorer diet, such as lower fruit and vegetable consumption [28], greater intake of soft drinks [29] and unhealthful sugary snacks [30]. Conversely, the relationship between overall sedentary time and cardiometabolic risk markers in children is less clear [10,31]. Screen-time, which current public health guidelines recommend children spend no more than two hours per day engaged in [32], may therefore have a stronger link with health due to its associations with numerous unhealthy lifestyle factors [15,33].

Previous studies investigating the relationship between screen-time and other lifestyle factors have solely focused on television (TV) viewing [30,34,35], which, given the vast array of available screen-based technologies, is no longer representative of modern society. Moreover, evidence investigating activity behaviours and diet in children has mainly concentrated on screen-time rather than PA, for which data, specifically amongst British children, is limited. Whilst some studies have investigated relationships between lifestyle factors and MVPA or screen-time, these have been conducted in isolation. Assessing both relationships simultaneously will not only enable a better understanding of the associated multiple lifestyle factors, but inform future interventions.

Therefore, the present study sought to explore associations between multiple lifestyle factors and being sufficiently active ($\geq$60 min·day^{-1}) or engaging in excessive screen-time ($\geq$2 h·day^{-1}) in children.

2. Materials and Methods

2.1. Participants

Data were captured on children who participated in the Swan-Linx programme, a health and fitness initiative, which is a sister project to Sportslinx [36,37]. In total, 756 children (371 boys, 385 girls) aged 9–11 years (10.4 $\pm$ 0.6 years) participated in the study. Data were collected across 13 socio-demographically representative schools ((WIMD: Welsh index of multiple deprivation) [38]), within the city and county of Swansea between January and May 2015. The Swan-Linx programme has University ethical approval for its procedures and measures. Head teacher and parental consent and child assent were obtained prior to data collection.

2.2. Instruments and Procedures

Anthropometric measurements were obtained using standard anthropometric techniques [39], by the same trained researcher. Children had their stature and body mass measured to the nearest 0.001 m and 0.1 kg, using a portable stadiometer (Seca 213 portable stadiometer, Hamburg, Germany) and electronic weighing scales (Seca 876, Hamburg, Germany), respectively. From these measures, Body Mass Index (BMI) was calculated (BMI = body mass (kg)/stature^2 (m)) and BMI z-scores were derived using the British 1990 growth reference standard [40]. The 20 metre multi-stage fitness test (20 MSFT) [41], which has been shown to be valid and reliable in similarly-aged children [42], was conducted by the same trained researchers using a standardised lap scoring protocol [43] to assess cardiorespiratory fitness. Both the anthropometric measurements and 20 MSFT were carried out at the indoor training centre at Swansea University.

Participants were asked to complete an online 29-item lifestyle questionnaire (CHAT: Child Health and Activity Tool) akin to the paper-based tool used in Sportlinx [44]. The CHAT questionnaire assessed time spent in MVPA, homework/reading and screen-time, as well as dietary habits, age and sleep duration. The description of screen-time included time spent watching TV, playing computer games and tablet/internet use, whereas MVPA was defined as "any activity or sport where your heart beats faster, you breathed faster and you felt warmer". Participants were asked to report time spent in each activity before (8 categories ranging from "no time at all" to "more than 1 hour") and after-school (10 categories ranging from "no time at all" to "more than 3 hours"). There were also questions asking the children how many days a week they engaged in excessive screen-time ($\geq$2 h·day^{-1}) and were sufficiently active ($\geq$60 min·day^{-1}). Further, participants were asked how many portions of fruit and vegetables they had consumed the previous day, whether they had breakfast, and how many days of the week they had at least one of the following: a takeaway meal, a sugary snack, a full sugar soft drink or a diet soft drink. Participants were asked to report the time they went to sleep and woke up, from which sleep duration was calculated and split into seven groups (<5.5 h; 5.5–6.4 h; 6.5–7.4 h; 7.5–9.4 h; 9.5–11.9 h; 12–12.9 h; 13–14.5 h). Participants postcodes (i.e., zip codes) were collected to calculate a WIMD score, which considers eight domains of deprivation; employment; health; income; housing; community safety; access to services; education and the environment [38].

2.3. Statistical Analysis

Missing data were noted for BMI (8 boys (2.2%), 29 girls (7.5%)), CRF (20 boys (5.4%), 22 girls (5.9%)), dietary and activity behaviours (11 boys (3%), 12 girls (3.1%)) and sleep duration (16 boys (4.3%), 18 girls (4.7%)). Statistical analyses were completed using IBM SPSS statistics 22 (IBM SPSS Statistics Inc., Chicago, IL, USA), where significance was set at $\leq$0.05. Whilst the normality assumption was violated, research suggests that it is not necessary when the sample size is large (>200) [45,46], therefore parametric tests were deemed appropriate. Multi-collinearity diagnostics were applied to all the variables. Linear regression models, were used to examine the extent to which the lifestyle factors (BMI z-scores; CRF; screen-time, homework/reading and MVPA before and after school; fruit and vegetable consumption; breakfast consumption; full sugar soft drink intake; diet soft drink intake; sugary snack consumption; sleep duration and takeaway meal consumption) and potential confounders (i.e., WIMD and age) predicted the number of days a week in excessive screen-time and in sufficient levels of MVPA. Variables with a significant result ($p < 0.10$) were added to a multiple regression model using the backward elimination approach. Variables that were not significant ($p > 0.10$) were deleted in a stepwise manner, resulting in a model with only significant interactions ($p < 0.05$). An independent t-test and a χ^2 test for the continuous and categorical variables, respectively, revealed significant differences between boys and girls and therefore regression models were conducted separately by sex. For each sex, the dependent variables were split at the median to form high and low screen-time and MVPA groups. Cut-off points of $\geq$5 and $\geq$4 days in sufficient MVPA for boys and girls respectively, were used to create MVPA groups. To classify screen-time groups, cut-off points of $\geq$4 and $\geq$3 days in excessive screen-time for boys and girls respectively were used. To help facilitate the interpretation of the different associations between the independent and dependent variables, differences between the high and low groups were tested post hoc using independent t-tests and χ^2 tests for continuous and categorical variables, respectively.

3. Results

Descriptive statistics for the original data set are presented in Table 1. Boys had significantly higher CRF ($p < 0.01$) compared with girls, and engaged in more screen-time before ($p < 0.01$) and afterschool ($p < 0.01$). Furthermore, boys had higher full sugar soft drink consumption ($p = 0.01$), spent more time in MVPA after school ($p = 0.04$), and consumed less fruit and vegetables ($p = 0.02$). Breakfast was consumed by 94.1% of the children (93.6% boys, 94.6% girls). There were no significant sex differences for the number of days a week spent in excessive screen-time [32] or in sufficient levels of MVPA [23].

Models showing significant associations between the lifestyle factors, being sufficiently active and excessive screen-time are shown in Table 2. Among boys, time spent in MVPA ($p < 0.01$) and homework/reading after school ($p = 0.05$), CRF ($p < 0.01$) and fruit and vegetable consumption ($p < 0.01$) were positively associated with being sufficiently active. Excessive screen-time was positively associated with screen-time after-school ($p < 0.01$), diet soft drink intake ($p = 0.03$) and sugary snack consumption ($p < 0.01$) and negatively associated with MVPA before school ($p = 0.01$).

For girls, being sufficiently active was positively associated with MVPA after school ($p < 0.01$), CRF ($p = 0.02$) and fruit and vegetable consumption ($p < 0.01$) and negatively associated with takeaway meals ($p = 0.01$). Further, screen-time after school ($p < 0.01$) and sugary snack consumption ($p < 0.01$) were positively associated, whereas MVPA before school ($p = 0.01$), sleep duration ($p = 0.03$) and fruit and vegetable consumption ($p = 0.01$) were negatively associated with excessive screen-time.

Descriptive characteristics for the high vs. low groups are presented in Table 3. Post hoc analyses revealed that, irrespective of sex, children in the high PA groups had higher CRF ($p < 0.01$), consumed more fruit and vegetables ($p < 0.01$) and spent more time in MVPA before and after school ($p < 0.01$). Girls in the low PA group consumed more takeaway meals ($p < 0.01$) and had higher screen-time before school ($p = 0.04$). Regarding screen-time, girls and boys in the high group had lower CRF ($p = 0.02$ girls, $p = 0.01$ boys), consumed more full sugar ($p < 0.01$) and diet soft drinks ($p = 0.02$ girls, $p < 0.01$ boys) and consumed more sugary snacks ($p < 0.01$).

Furthermore, both sexes in the high screen-time groups consumed more takeaway meals ($p = 0.04$ girls, $p = 0.01$ boys), had higher screen-time before and after school ($p < 0.01$) and spent less time in MVPA before school ($p < 0.01$ girls, $p = 0.01$ boys). Moreover, girls in the high screen-time group consumed less fruit and vegetables ($p < 0.01$), while boys in this group spent less time in MVPA after school ($p = 0.01$). Although, the number of takeaway meals ($p < 0.01$) and CRF levels ($p = 0.02$ girls, $p < 0.01$ boys) were significantly associated with excessive screen-time in both sexes when examined separately, the associations were no longer significant in the final regression model after controlling for confounders. In addition, despite diet ($p = 0.01$) and full sugar soft drink intake ($p < 0.01$) being univariately associated with excessive screen-time in girls and boys, respectively, these associations did not remain significant after controlling for other confounders.

Table 1. Descriptive data.

Characteristics	Total Sample (n = 756)		Boys (n = 371)		Girls (n = 385)		
	Mean (SD)	n	Mean (SD)	n	Mean (SD)	n	P
Age (years)	10.4 (0.6)	752	10.4 (0.6)	369	10.4 (0.6)	383	0.96
WIMD	850.1 (571.1)	756	819.5 (578.7)	371	879.7 (562.8)	385	0.15
Height (cm)	142.1 (7.8)	731	141.8 (7.4)	366	142.0 (8.2)	365	0.21
Body mass (kg)	38.6 (10.2)	724	38.0 (10.5)	365	39.3 (9.9)	360	0.78
BMI	18.9 (3.8)	723	18.7 (3.8)	365	19.2 (3.7)	358	0.08
BMI z-score	0.6 (1.3)	719	0.6 (1.3)	363	0.6 (1.3)	356	0.06
CRF (No. of shuttles run)	31.0 (16.4)	700	36.3 (18.2)	351	25.6 (12.4)	349	<0.01 *
No. of days a week being sufficiently active	4.4 (2.2)	733	4.4 (2.3)	360	4.4 (2.0)	373	0.97
No. of days a week in excessive screen-time	3.7 (2.4)	733	3.9 (2.4)	360	3.6 (2.4)	373	0.14
No. of days a week drinking at least one full sugar soft drink	1.9 (2.1)	733	2.1 (2.3)	360	1.7 (2.0)	373	0.01 *
No. of days a week drinking at least one diet soft drink	1.3 (2.0)	733	1.4 (2.0)	360	1.3 (1.9)	373	0.28
No. of fruit and vegetable portions eaten yesterday	3.2 (1.9)	731	3.0 (2.0)	360	3.4 (1.8)	371	0.02 *
No. of days a week eating at least one sugary snack	3.2 (1.9)	733	3.2 (2.2)	360	3.2 (2.0)	373	0.71
No. of days a week eating at least one takeaway meal	1.0 (1.3)	733	1.0 (1.4)	360	1.0 (1.3)	373	0.53
MVPA before school (min)	14.2 (15.5)	733	14.6 (15.7)	360	14.0 (15.2)	733	0.16
MVPA after school (min)	54.1 (55.5)	732	60.3 (60.7)	360	48.0 (49.2)	732	0.04 *
Homework/reading before school (min)	10.4 (13.8)	733	10.4 (13.8)	360	10.0 (13.8)	373	1.00
Homework/reading after school (min)	17.7 (25.8)	732	16.2 (25.9)	360	19.0 (25.6)	372	0.12
Screen-time before school (min)	14.0 (18.7)	733	17.1 (20.2)	360	11.0 (16.6)	373	<0.01 *
Screen-time after school (min)	45.1 (52.1)	732	55.7 (59.0)	360	35.0 (41.9)	372	<0.01 *
Sleep duration (h)	9.8 (1.3)	723	9.8 (1.5)	354	9.9 (1.2)	367	0.35

p-Values are based on significance level from the independent t-test for continuous variables (non-italics) or the chi-squared test for categorical variables (italics). * Relationship is significant. BMI: body mass index; CRF: cardio-respiratory fitness; MVPA: moderate-to-vigorous intensity physical activity; WIMD: welsh index of multiple deprivation.

Table 2. Multiple regression models conducted separately by sex.

Model	Predictors	Boys (n = 371)			Girls (n = 385)		
		B (SE)	β	P	B (SE)	β	P
No. of days being sufficiently active	MVPA before school (min)	-	-	-	0.01 (0.01)	0.09	0.06
	MVPA after school (min)	0.01 (0.00)	0.38	<0.01*	0.01 (0.00)	0.35	<0.01*
	Homework/reading after school (min)	0.01 (0.00)	0.09	0.05*	-	-	-
	CRF (No. of shuttles run)	0.03 (0.01)	0.20	<0.01*	0.02 (0.01)	0.11	0.02*
	No. of days a week eating at least one takeaway meal	-	-	-	-0.20 (0.07)	-0.13	0.01*
	No. of fruit and vegetable portions eaten yesterday	0.27 (0.05)	0.25	<0.01*	0.27 (0.06)	0.24	<0.01*
	R^2 (adjusted R^2)		0.35 (0.34)			0.30 (0.29)	
No. of days in excessive screen-time	MVPA before school (min)	-0.02 (0.01)	-0.12	0.01*	-0.02 (0.01)	-0.13	0.01*
	Homework/reading before school (min)	-0.01 (0.01)	-0.08	0.08	-	-	-
	Screen-time before school (min)	0.03 (0.01)	0.22	<0.01*	0.03 (0.01)	0.18	<0.01*
	Screen-time after school (min)	0.02 (0.00)	0.35	<0.01*	0.02 (0.00)	0.27	<0.01*
	No. of fruit and vegetable portions eaten yesterday	-	-	-	-0.17 (0.07)	-0.12	0.01*
	No. of days a week drinking at least one diet drink	0.11 (0.05)	0.09	0.03*	-	-	-
	No. of days a week drinking at least one full sugar soft drink	-	-	-	0.12 (0.60)	0.10	0.05*
	No. of days a week eating at least one sugary snack	0.17 (0.05)	0.16	<0.01*	0.18 (0.06)	0.15	<0.01*
	Age	-	-	-	0.37 (0.19)	0.09	0.05*
	Sleep duration	-	-	-	-0.36 (0.17)	-0.10	0.03*
	R^2 (adjusted R^2)		0.41 (0.40)			0.33 (0.32)	

CRF: Cardio-respiratory fitness; MVPA: moderate-to-vigorous intensity physical activity. * Relationship is significant.

Table 3. Descriptive statistics for the high and low screen-time and MVPA groups.

Characteristics	Boys (n = 371)						Girls (n = 386)					
	Low MVPA (n = 165)	High MVPA (n = 195)	P	Low Screen-Time (n = 187)	High Screen-Time (n = 173)	P	Low MVPA (n = 137)	High MVPA (n = 236)	P	Low Screen-Time (n = 141)	High Screen-Time (n = 232)	P
	Mean (SD)	Mean (SD)		Mean (SD)	Mean (SD)		Mean (SD)	Mean (SD)		Mean (SD)	Mean (SD)	
Age (years)	10.4 (0.6)	10.4 (0.6)	0.16	10.4 (0.6)	10.4 (0.6)	0.27	10.3 (0.6)	10.5 (0.6)	<0.01*	10.3 (0.6)	10.5 (0.6)	0.08
WIMD	799.0 (578.9)	834.9 (580.4)	0.56	917.1 (576.6)	771.9 (564.4)	<0.01*	872.3 (546.5)	885.8 (574.2)	0.82	916.0 (566.4)	859.4 (561.8)	0.35
Height (cm)	141.1 (7.8)	142.4 (7.2)	0.10	141.7 (6.9)	141.9 (8.1)	0.84	140.8 (8.3)	143.4 (8.1)	<0.01*	141.6 (8.2)	142.9 (8.2)	0.16
Body mass (kg)	37.8 (11.0)	38.4 (10.3)	0.57	37.9 (9.4)	38.4 (11.8)	0.68	38.3 (10.5)	40.1 (9.7)	0.09	38.5 (9.3)	40.0 (10.0)	0.16
BMI	18.7 (3.8)	18.7 (3.8)	0.93	18.7 (3.5)	18.8 (4.1)	0.79	19.2 (4.2)	19.3 (3.5)	0.65	19.0 (3.5)	19.4 (3.9)	0.29
BMI z-score	0.6 (1.4)	0.6 (1.3)	0.98	0.7 (1.2)	0.6 (1.4)	0.58	0.5 (1.5)	0.6 (1.1)	0.40	0.5 (1.2)	0.6 (1.3)	0.53
CRF (No. of shuttles run)	30.1 (14.8)	41.1 (19.4)	<0.01*	38.7 (18.7)	33.2 (17.4)	0.01*	22.5 (10.4)	27.2 (13.2)	<0.01*	27.6 (13.7)	24.1 (11.3)	0.02*
No. of days a week being sufficiently active	2.3 (1.3)	6.3 (0.9)	<0.01*	4.6 (2.2)	4.3 (2.4)	0.25	2.2 (0.9)	5.7 (1.2)	<0.01*	4.5 (2.1)	4.4 (2.0)	0.44
No. of days a week in excessive screen-time	4.1 (2.5)	3.7 (2.4)	0.10	1.8 (1.0)	6.2 (1.1)	<0.01*	3.7 (2.5)	3.5 (2.3)	0.40	1.1 (0.8)	5.1 (1.6)	<0.01*
No. of days a week drinking at least one full sugar soft drink	2.1 (2.2)	2.1 (2.3)	0.93	1.5 (1.9)	2.8 (2.5)	<0.01*	1.9 (2.0)	1.6 (2.0)	0.17	1.2 (1.6)	2.0 (2.2)	<0.01*
No. of days a week drinking at least one diet soft drink	1.4 (2.0)	1.4 (2.1)	0.93	1.1 (1.6)	1.8 (2.4)	<0.01*	1.3 (1.9)	1.2 (1.9)	0.69	1.0 (1.6)	1.4 (2.0)	0.02*
No. of fruit and vegetable portions eaten yesterday	2.3 (1.8)	3.7 (2.0)	<0.01*	3.2 (2.0)	2.8 (2.1)	0.06	2.7 (1.6)	3.8 (1.8)	<0.01*	3.8 (1.8)	3.1 (1.7)	<0.01*
No. of days a week eating at least one sugary snack	3.2 (2.3)	3.3 (2.2)	0.56	2.4 (1.8)	4.1 (2.4)	<0.01*	3.2 (2.0)	3.2 (2.1)	0.93	2.5 (1.7)	3.6 (2.1)	<0.01*
No. of days a week eating at least one takeaway meal	1.0 (1.4)	1.1 (1.3)	0.51	0.9 (1.1)	1.2 (1.6)	0.01*	1.2 (1.5)	0.8 (1.2)	<0.01*	0.8 (1.3)	1.1 (1.3)	0.04*
MVPA before school (min)	9.6 (12.5)	18.9 (16.9)	<0.01*	17.7 (17.4)	11.3 (13.1)	0.01*	10.7 (14.5)	15.4 (15.1)	<0.01*	17.9 (16.7)	11.1 (13.3)	<0.01*

Table 3. Cont.

Characteristics	Boys (n = 371)						Girls (n = 386)					
	Low MVPA (n = 163)	High MVPA (n = 195)		Low Screen-Time (n = 187)	High Screen-Time (n = 173)		Low MVPA (n = 137)	High MVPA (n = 236)		Low Screen-Time (n = 141)	High Screen-Time (n = 232)	
MVPA after school (min)	32.2 (42.7)	84.0 (63.5)	<0.01 *	69.8 (62.2)	49.9 (57.4)	0.01 *	25.4 (31.2)	61.5 (53.0)	<0.01 *	55.6 (50.2)	43.7 (48.3)	0.24
Homework/reading before school (min)	8.4 (11.9)	12.2 (14.9)	0.08	11.6 (14.5)	9.2 (12.9)	0.35	8.8 (12.6)	11.3 (14.4)	0.70	12.5 (14.6)	9.1 (13.2)	0.20
Homework/reading after school (min)	12.7 (20.7)	19.1 (29.4)	0.25	16.5 (23.4)	15.9 (28.4)	0.81	14.7 (16.9)	21.8 (29.3)	0.39	19.4 (20.5)	19.1 (28.3)	0.53
Screen-time before school (min)	18.8 (21.0)	15.7 (19.4)	0.72	9.9 (13.9)	24.8 (22.9)	<0.01 *	14.3 (18.9)	9.1 (15.0)	0.04 *	5.4 (11.6)	14.4 (18.4)	<0.01 *
Screen-time after school (min)	61.2 (62.1)	51.0 (56.0)	0.21	28.9 (38.1)	84.6 (63.9)	<0.01 *	41.5 (47.0)	31.1 (38.4)	0.29	17.0 (26.5)	45.9 (45.9)	<0.01 *
Sleep duration (h)	9.7 (1.5)	9.8 (1.4)	0.55	9.9 (1.3)	9.6 (1.6)	0.11	9.9 (1.2)	10.0 (1.2)	0.97	10.1 (1.2)	9.8 (1.2)	0.12

p-Values are based on significance level from the independent t-test for continuous variables (non-italics) or the chi-squared test for categorical variables (italics). * Relationship is significant. BMI: body mass index; CRF: Cardio-respiratory fitness; MVPA: moderate-to-vigorous intensity physical activity; WIMD: welsh index of multiple deprivation. The cut-off value for MVPA was $\geq$5 and $\geq$4 days in sufficient MVPA for boys and girls respectively. The cut-off value for screen time was $\geq$4 and $\geq$3 days in excessive screen-time for boys and girls respectively.

4. Discussion

The present study aimed to explore associations between MVPA, sedentary time and multiple lifestyle factors in 9–11 years old children. Of note, there was no inverse relationship between days spent in excessive screen-time and sufficient levels of MVPA or vice versa. Although studies have reported an inverse relationship between sedentary time and MVPA [47], there is insufficient evidence to assume a reciprocal relationship [47]. Whilst both behaviours may directly compete with each other during a specific time period (e.g., after school) [47], the same may not be true for an entire day or across a week [48]. Further, similar to previous research [15,25,29,49], excessive screen-time was associated with unhealthy factors, which were different to those inversely related to sufficient levels of MVPA. Indeed, available evidence suggests that they are two separate entities [9], which are independently associated with health [10].

While boys were more active than girls after school, both were sufficiently active for the same number of days a week. Consistent with a recent review [7], sufficient levels of MVPA were positively related to CRF independent of sex. Aside from low CRF, low fruit and vegetable intake is another weight-related risk factor [11]. In agreement with previous research [15,16,50], strong positive associations between fruit and vegetable consumption and sufficient levels of MVPA were observed in both sexes. Conversely, Pereira et al. [51] found a negative relationship, whereas Vissers et al. [52] and Jago et al. [53] found a positive relationship in boys and girls, respectively. The equivocal findings may, in part, be a result of different methodologies and sample characteristics; Pereira et al. [51] found active children engaged in more screen-time, and studies have suggested a negative relationship between screen-time and fruit and vegetable consumption [29,49]; in contrast to the present study, Vissers et al. [52] found MVPA to be significantly higher in boys and Jago et al. [53] recorded dietary and PA measures 12 months apart.

Sleep duration is an important component of health in children [9] and has been associated with MVPA, however evidence is scarce and contradictory. In our study, sufficient levels of MVPA were not associated with sleep duration. On the contrary, Stone et al. [14] found MVPA to be higher among children with >10 h of sleep per night compared with those who slept <9 h per night. However, it is noteworthy that Stone et al. [14] used parental report to assess sleep duration, which is thought to have questionable reliability, as parents tend to overestimate sleep duration [54,55]. Although children can also overestimate sleep duration [56], our finding that sleep duration was not associated with MVPA is in agreement with several studies that measured sleep duration objectively [21,57]. In children of this age, sleep duration may be more susceptible to environmental factors, such as social activities or school arrangements than the actual need for sleep [57], which may explain why MVPA was not directly associated. However, MVPA has been associated with better sleep efficiency [57,58] and shorter sleep latency [57] and is therefore considered beneficial for sleep in children.

Converse to a systematic review [59], this study did not find an association between BMI and sufficient levels of MVPA irrespective of sex. There was a large amount of data missing for BMI in girls (7.5%); although the weight status of these girls is unknown, it is possible that they were overweight or obese. The extent to which this biased results is unclear, however it may provide a reason for why there was no association between BMI and MVPA in girls. Further, this relationship may be more related to the intensity of PA as opposed to total PA [60]; therefore the aggregation of moderate (MPA) and vigorous (VPA) physical activity may, in part, explain this discrepancy.

The lack of association between excessive screen-time and BMI-z scores in the present study, may have been due to the low prevalence of reported screen-time in the sample. On average, children engaged in ≥2 hours of screen-time for only 3.7 days a week, compared with the average of 3 hours per day reported in studies observing a relationship between screen-time and adiposity in children [12,61]. Therefore, perhaps only higher durations of screen-time are associated with adiposity in children [10]. Although the underpinning mechanisms behind the relationship between screen-time and adiposity are not completely understood [10], the association between screen-time and elements of a less healthy diet is believed to be a contributing factor [29]. Sugary snack consumption was positively associated with excessive screen-time in this study, in agreement with previous research [28,29,49]. As sugary snack consumption has been shown to increase overall caloric intake [8], it may be an important factor in the screen-time and obesity/overweight relationship. Screen-time may influence sugary snack consumption in children in several ways, through exposure to advertisements for sugary snacks on TV or online [62], reduced sensitivity to satiety cues and messages imbedded in TV programmes [63]. Interestingly, diet soft drinks are the most highly advertised product on TV [62], and since boys watch more TV [33,64], they are more exposed to these advertisements which may explain the positive relationship between diet soft drinks and excessive screen-time in boys.

For girls only, low fruit and vegetable consumption was associated with screen time, consistent with a recent review by Pearson and Biddle [49]. It is not clear why the relationship only exists in girls, but it may be partially explained by the positive but non-significant relationship between sufficient levels of MVPA and excessive screen-time in boys ($p = 0.08$). Similarly, others have also found high levels of MVPA and screen-time to co-exist in boys [65,66]. Therefore, fruit and vegetable consumption may be higher among boys who engage in excessive screen time as they are also achieving sufficient levels of MVPA, since a positive relationship exists between the latter and fruit and vegetable consumption.

In contrast to previous research [25,26], we observed a negative relationship between screen-time and sleep duration only in girls. The reason for this sex difference is not clear, but mobile phone and MP3 player use is higher among girls, whereas watching TV and video gaming is higher among boys [64]. As mobile phones and MP3 players are easier to hide from parents in bed [67], it could be postulated that the more frequent use of these devices by girls before bedtime could reduce sleep time.

The negative relationship observed between MVPA before school and excessive screen-time may reflect findings from Gorely et al. [68] whereby adolescents who commuted to school via motorised transport were more likely to spend their discretionary time watching screens. Since active travel is considered the main source of MVPA before school [36], it is possible that children who engaged in excessive screen-time commuted to and from school via motorised transport. However, since few studies have investigated associations between active travel to school and screen-time in children to date, more research is needed to confirm the potential influence of active travel on habitual screen-time.

We found positive associations between MVPA and screen-time after-school and meeting and exceeding their respective recommendations, respectively, which supports the hypothesis that the after-school period is key for the accumulation of MVPA and screen-time [36]. Indeed, Atkin et al. [24] revealed that time spent in both screen-time and MVPA during the after-school period (15:30–18:30) accounted for approximately 30% and 40%, respectively, of daily totals. Further, Olds et al. [27] found that during this period the greatest variation in MVPA levels occurred between high active and low active children.

Although screen-time and MVPA are the most prominent behaviours during the after-school period [24,69], productive sedentary behaviours, such as homework and reading, also occur and are thought to directly compete with MVPA [70]. However, in the present study, there was a positive relationship between homework/reading after school and sufficient levels of MVPA in boys, similar to data reported in adolescents [71]. In accord with Booth et al. [19], this suggests that there is time for both MVPA and homework and reading throughout the day and provides support for the beneficial influence of MVPA on school endeavours in boys at least. In contrast to most types of screen-based sedentary behaviours, these productive sedentary behaviours are considered essential for a child's education and development [9].

The present study has numerous strengths. Firstly, to the authors' knowledge, it is the first study to investigate the associations of both sufficient levels of MVPA and excessive screen-time with multiple lifestyle factors in children within the same sample. The integration of new types of technology for assessing screen-time advances previous research, which focused solely on television viewing [30,34,35]. This is important as screen-time is constantly changing due to technological advances, and multifunctional devices such as tablets, smartphones and computers are now frequently used by children [64]. Moreover, children regularly engage in two or more forms of screen viewing simultaneously [72]. Therefore, children can over-report screen-time when responding to certain self-report questions, however we were able to address this with our excessive screen-time question. Further, the sample was socio-demographically representative of the area and the detailed information collected enabled us to control for a number of variables. Also, while there is sufficient research investigating associations between diet and MVPA in adults [73] and adolescents [74], there is a paucity of research among children. In addition, the present study established a number of sex differences in relationships, uncommon in the literature. These may be a function of measurement issues, but equally, they may just be sample dependent, differing by cultural environments, age or country of study.

Nonetheless, certain limitations should be acknowledged. Given the cross-sectional nature of the study, it is not possible to infer causal relationships and future research should clarify such complex relationships by examining longitudinal associations. In addition, the time-specific measures used to assess diet, MVPA, screen-time and sleep duration may not have captured habitual behaviour. Future studies should seek to assess diet [28,52] and screen-time [75] using 7 day diary/logs and similarly PA [13] and sleep duration [76] for 7 days by accelerometer. Measuring PA using an accelerometer also allows researchers to quantify intensity, which the questionnaire did not allow as it primarily focused on the frequency and duration of PA. Indeed, MPA and VPA were aggregated, and VPA is more consistently associated with health [7]. Moreover, the comparably low prevalence of excessive screen-time found in the sample may be due, at least in part, to social desirability, inherent in self-reporting [75]. Unfortunately, as the screen-time measure is an aggregate of three behaviours, we could not examine TV viewing, playing computer games and tablet/internet use separately. There is evidence to suggest that internet use for productive purposes, is not related to poor lifestyle habits in adolescents [77]. Even internet use for gaming may have less of an impact on poor lifestyle habits, such as snacking than TV viewing, particularly in boys [78]. Direct comparisons between this cross-sectional study and others are limited by the different study designs and methodologies used to assess behaviours. Whilst, previous studies examining multiple lifestyle factors have used approaches such as cluster and co-occurrence analyses [51,79], this is one of the few to explore the independent associations between MVPA, screen-time and several other lifestyle factors, while simultaneously controlling for potential confounders. The approach utilized in the present study enabled the identification of several important lifestyle factors, which could be beneficially influenced through implementing interventions designed to change MVPA and screen-time. As such, the study is of significant public health interest.

5. Conclusions

Taken together, the present study enables researchers to gain a better understanding of other lifestyle factors associated with MVPA and screen-time in children. Specifically, both healthy and unhealthy lifestyle factors, differing by sex, were associated with sufficient levels of MVPA and excessive screen-time respectively. Future interventions seeking to promote health behaviours, should target change in multiple lifestyle factors, with sex-specific strategies. Further, the home environment is recognised to have a large influence on lifestyle factors in children, particularly on sedentary time and MVPA [80]. Therefore, research exploring lifestyle correlates of MVPA and sedentary time within this environment is needed.

Acknowledgments: The authors wish to thank the schools, the children and their parents for their participation in the Swan-Linx programme. The authors would also like to acknowledge everyone who helped with data collection. Michael Sheldrick is supported by a Zienkiewicz scholarship awarded by Swansea University.

Author Contributions: Michael P. R. Sheldrick analysed the data and wrote the manuscript. Richard Tyler collected the data, assembled the input data and edited the manuscript. Gareth Stratton and Kelly A. Mackintosh supervised the analyses and edited the manuscript.

Conflicts of Interest: The authors declare no conflict of interest.

References

1. Karnik, S.; Kanekar, A.A. Childhood Obesity: A Global Public Health Crisis. *Int. J. Prev. Med.* **2012**, 1, 1–7. [CrossRef]
2. Jones, M.; Blackaby, D.; Murphy, P. Childhood Obesity in Wales. *Welsh Econ. Rev.* **2006**, 22, 36–42.
3. Singh, A.S.; Mulder, C.; Twisk, J.W.R.; Van Mechelen, W.; Chinapaw, M.J.M. Tracking of childhood overweight into adulthood: A systematic review of the literature. *Obes. Rev.* **2008**, 9, 474–488. [CrossRef] [PubMed]
4. Bridger, T. Childhood obesity and cardiovascular disease. *Paediatr. Child Health* **2009**, 14, 177–182. [CrossRef] [PubMed]
5. Pulgaron, E.R.; Delamater, A.M. Obesity and type 2 diabetes in children: Epidemiology and treatment. *Curr. Diab. Rep.* **2014**, 14, 1–21. [CrossRef] [PubMed]
6. Biro, F.M.; Wien, M. Childhood obesity and adult morbidities. *Am. J. Clin. Nutr.* **2010**, 91, 1499–1505. [CrossRef]
7. Poitras, V.J.; Gray, C.E.; Borghese, M.M.; Carson, V.; Chaput, J.; Janssen, I.; Katzmarzyk, P.T.; Pate, R.R.; Gorber, S.C.; Kho, M.E.; et al. Systematic review of the relationships between objectively measured physical activity and health indicators in school-aged children and youth. *Appl. Physiol. Nutr. Metab.* **2016**, 239. [CrossRef] [PubMed]
8. Bhadoria, A.; Sahoo, K.; Sahoo, B.; Choudhury, A.; Sufi, N.; Kumar, R. Childhood obesity: Causes and consequences. *J. Fam. Med. Prim. Care* **2015**, 4, 187. [CrossRef] [PubMed]
9. Carson, V.; Tremblay, M.S.; Chaput, J.-P.; Chastin, S.F.; Carson, V.; Tremblay, M.; Chaput, J.; Chastin, S. Associations between sleep duration, sedentary time, physical activity, and health indicators among Canadian children and youth using compositional analyses 1. *Appl. Physiol. Nutr. Metab.* **2016**, 41, 294–302. [CrossRef] [PubMed]
10. Carson, V.; Hunter, S.; Kuzik, N.; Gray, C.E.; Poitras, V.J.; Chaput, J.-P.; Saunders, T.J.; Katzmarzyk, P.T.; Okely, A.D.; Connor Gorber, S.; et al. Systematic review of sedentary behaviour and health indicators in school-aged children and youth: An update 1. *Appl. Physiol. Nutr. Metab.* **2016**, 41, 240–265. [CrossRef] [PubMed]
11. Ledoux, T.A.; Hingle, M.D.; Baranowski, T. Relationship of fruit and vegetable intake with adiposity: A systematic review. *Obes. Rev.* **2011**, 12, 143–150. [CrossRef] [PubMed]
12. Wilkie, H.J.; Standage, M.; Gillison, F.B.; Cumming, S.P.; Katzmarzyk, P.T. Multiple lifestyle behaviours and overweight and obesity among children aged 9–11 years: Results from the UK site of the International Study of Childhood Obesity, Lifestyle and the Environment. *BMJ Open* **2016**, 6, e010677. [CrossRef] [PubMed]
13. Katzmarzyk, P.T.; Barreira, T.V.; Broyles, S.T.; Champagne, C.M.; Chaput, J.P.; Fogelholm, M.; Hu, G.; Johnson, W.D.; Kuriyan, R.; Kurpad, A.; et al. Physical Activity, Sedentary Time, and Obesity in an International Sample of Children. *Med. Sci. Sports Exerc.* **2015**, 47, 2062–2069. [CrossRef] [PubMed]
14. Stone, M.R.; Stevens, D.; Faulkner, G.E.J. Maintaining recommended sleep throughout the week is associated with increased physical activity in children. *Prev. Med.* **2013**, 56, 112–117. [CrossRef] [PubMed]
15. Lazzeri, G.; Azzolini, E.; Pammolli, A.; De Wet, D.R.; Giacchi, M.V. Correlation between physical activity and sedentary behavior with healthy and unhealthy behaviors in Italy and Tuscan region: A cross sectional study. *J. Prev. Med. Hyg.* **2013**, 54, 41–48. [PubMed]
16. Silva, D.A.S.; Silva, R.J.D.S. Association between physical activity level and consumption of fruit and vegetables among adolescents in northeast Brazil. *Rev. Paul. Pediatr.* **2015**, 33, 167–173. [CrossRef] [PubMed]
17. Pearson, N.; Atkin, A.J.; Biddle, S.J.; Gorely, T.; Edwardson, C. Patterns of adolescent physical activity and dietary behaviours. *Int. J. Behav. Nutr. Phys. Act.* **2009**, 6, 45. [CrossRef] [PubMed]
18. Szczerbiński, R.; Karczewski, J.K.; Siemienkowicz, J. Selected Nourishment Habits Depending on Physical Activity of 14-16 Year-Old Teenagers in the North-Eastern Poland on the Example of Sokolski District. *Rocz. Panstw. Zaki. Hig.* **2010**, 61, 83–86.
19. Booth, J.N.; Leary, S.D.; Joinson, C.; Ness, A.R.; Tomporowski, P.D.; Boyle, J.M.; Reilly, J.J. Associations between objectively measured physical activity and academic attainment in adolescents from a UK cohort. *Br. J. Sports Med.* **2014**, 48, 265–270. [CrossRef] [PubMed]
20. Sjödin, A.; Hjorth, M.F.; Damsgaard, C.T.; Ritz, C.; Astrup, A.; Michaelsen, K.F. Physical activity, sleep duration and metabolic health in children fluctuate with the lunar cycle: Science behind the myth. *Clin. Obes.* **2015**, 5, 60–66. [CrossRef] [PubMed]

21. Mcneil, J.; Tremblay, M.S.; Leduc, G.; Boyer, C.; Bélanger, P.; Leblanc, A.G.; Borghese, M.M.; Chaput, J.P. Objectively-measured sleep and its association with adiposity and physical activity in a sample of Canadian children. *J. Sleep Res.* **2015**, *24*, 131–139. [CrossRef] [PubMed]

22. Vaisto, J.; Eloranta, A.M.; Viitasalo, A.; Tompuri, T.; Lintu, N.; Karjalainen, P.; Lampinen, E.K.; Agren, J.; Laaksonen, D.E.; Lakka, H.M.; et al. Physical activity and sedentary behaviour in relation to cardiometabolic risk in children: Cross-sectional findings from the Physical Activity and Nutrition in Children (PANIC) Study. *Int. J. Behav. Nutr. Phys. Act.* **2014**, *11*, 55. [CrossRef] [PubMed]

23. Department of Health, Physical Activity, Health Improvement and Protection. *Start Active, Stay Active: A Report on Physical Activity for Health from the Four Home Countries' Chief Medical Officers*; Crown: London, UK, 2011.

24. Atkin, A.J.; Gorely, T.; Biddle, S.J.H.; Marshall, S.J.; Cameron, N. Critical hours: Physical activity and sedentary behavior of adolescents after school. *Pediatr. Exerc. Sci.* **2008**, *20*, 446–456. [CrossRef] [PubMed]

25. Hale, L.; Guan, S. Screen time and sleep among school-aged children and adolescents: A systematic literature review. *Sleep Med. Rev.* **2015**, *21*, 50–58. [CrossRef] [PubMed]

26. Falbe, J.; Davison, K.K.; Franckle, R.L.; Ganter, C.; Gortmaker, S.L.; Smith, L.; Land, T.; Taveras, E.M. Sleep Duration, Restfulness, and Screens in the Sleep Environment. *Pediatrics* **2015**, *135*, e367–e375. [CrossRef] [PubMed]

27. Olds, T.; Maher, C.A.; Ridley, K. The Place of Physical Activity in the Time Budgets of 10-to 13-Year-Old Australian Children. *J. Phys. Act. Health* **2011**, *8*, 548–557. [CrossRef] [PubMed]

28. Shang, L.; Wang, J.W.; O'Loughlin, J.; Tremblay, A.; Mathieu, M.È.; Henderson, M.; Gray-Donald, K. Screen time is associated with dietary intake in overweight Canadian children. *Prev. Med. Rep.* **2015**, *2*, 265–269. [CrossRef] [PubMed]

29. Börnhorst, C.; Wijnhoven, T.M.A.; Kunešová, M.; Yngve, A.; Rito, A.I.; Lissner, L.; Duleva, V.; Petrauskiene, A.; Breda, J. WHO European Childhood Obesity Surveillance Initiative: Associations between sleep duration, screen time and food consumption frequencies. *BMC Public Health* **2015**, *15*, 442. [CrossRef] [PubMed]

30. Hare-Bruun, H.; Nielsen, B.M.; Kristensen, P.L.; Møller, N.C.; Togo, P.; Heitmann, B.L. Television viewing, food preferences, and food habits among children: A prospective epidemiological study. *BMC Public Health* **2011**, *11*, 311. [CrossRef] [PubMed]

31. Saunders, T.J.; Chaput, J.P.; Tremblay, M.S. Sedentary behaviour as an emerging risk factor for cardiometabolic diseases in children and youth. *Can. J. Diabetes* **2014**, *38*, 53–61. [CrossRef] [PubMed]

32. Tremblay, M.S.; Carson, V.; Chaput, J.-P.; Connor Gorber, S.; Dinh, T.; Duggan, M.; Faulkner, G.; Gray, C.E.; Gruber, R.; Janson, K.; et al. Canadian 24-Hour Movement Guidelines for Children and Youth: An Integration of Physical Activity, Sedentary Behaviour, and Sleep. *Appl. Physiol. Nutr. Metab.* **2016**, *41*, S311–S327. [CrossRef] [PubMed]

33. LeBlanc, A.G.; Katzmarzyk, P.T.; Barreira, T.V.; Broyles, S.T.; Chaput, J.P.; Church, T.S.; Fogelholm, M.; Harrington, D.M.; Hu, G.; Kuriyan, R.; et al. Correlates of total sedentary time and screen time in 9–11 year-old children around the world: The international study of childhood obesity, lifestyle and the environment. *PLoS ONE* **2015**, *10*, 1–20. [CrossRef] [PubMed]

34. Pearson, N.; Biddle, S.J.H.; Williams, L.; Worsley, A.; Crawford, D.; Ball, K. Adolescent television viewing and unhealthy snack food consumption: The mediating role of home availability of unhealthy snack foods. *Public Health Nutr.* **2014**, *17*, 317–323. [CrossRef] [PubMed]

35. Mota, J.; Ribeiro, J.C.; Carvalho, J.; Santos, M.P.; Martins, J. Television viewing and changes in body mass index and cardiorespiratory fitness over a two-year period in school children. *Pediatr. Exerc. Sci.* **2010**, *22*, 245–253. [CrossRef] [PubMed]

36. Fairclough, S.J.; Beighle, A.; Erwin, H.; Ridgers, N.D. School day segmented physical activity patterns of high and low active children. *BMC Public Health* **2012**, *12*, 406. [CrossRef] [PubMed]

37. Stratton, G.; Canoy, D.; Boddy, L.M.; Taylor, S.R.; Hackett, A.F.; Buchan, I.E. Cardiorespiratory fitness and body mass index of 9–11-year-old English children: A serial cross-sectional study from 1998 to 2004. *Int. J. Obes.* **2007**, *31*, 1172–1178. [CrossRef] [PubMed]

38. Noble, M.; Wright, G.; Smith, G.; Dibben, C. Measuring multiple deprivation at the small-area level. *Environ. Plan. A* **2006**, *38*, 169–185. [CrossRef]

39. Lohman, T.G.; Roche, A.F.; Martorell, R. *Anthropometric Standardization Reference Manual*; Wiley: New York, NY, USA, 1992. [CrossRef]

40. Cole, T.J. Growth monitoring with the British 1990 growth reference. *Arch. Dis. Child.* **1997**, *76*, 47–49. [CrossRef] [PubMed]
41. Léger, L.A.; Mercier, D.; Gadoury, C.; Lambert, J. The multistage 20 metre shuttle run test for aerobic fitness. *J. Sports Sci.* **1988**, *6*, 93–101. [CrossRef] [PubMed]
42. Mayorga-vega, D.; Aguilar-soto, P.; Viciana, J. Criterion-Related Validity of the 20-M Shuttle Run Test for Estimating Cardiorespiratory Fitness: A Meta-Analysis. *J. Sports Sci. Med.* **2015**, *14*, 536–547. [PubMed]
43. Riddoch, C.J. *The Northern Ireland Health and Fitness Survey-1989: The Fitness, Physical Activity, Attitudes and Lifestyles of Northern Ireland Post-Primary School Children*; The Queen's University of Belfast: Belfast, UK, 1990.
44. Fairclough, S.J.; Boddy, L.M.; Hackett, A.F.; Stratton, G. Associations between children's socioeconomic status, weight status, and sex, with screen-based sedentary behaviours and sport participation. *Int. J. Pediatr. Obes.* **2009**, *4*, 299–305. [CrossRef] [PubMed]
45. Lumley, T.; Diehr, P.; Emerson, S.; Chen, L. The Importance of the Normality Assumption in Large Public Health Data Sets. *Annu. Rev. Public Health* **2002**, *23*, 151–169. [CrossRef] [PubMed]
46. Williams, M.; Grajales, C.A.G.; Kurkiewicz, D. Assumptions of multiple regression: Correcting two misconceptions. *Pract. Assess. Res. Eval.* **2013**, *18*, 1–14.
47. Pearson, N.; Braithwaite, R.E.; Biddle, S.J.H.; van Sluijs, E.M.F.; Atkin, A.J. Associations between sedentary behaviour and physical activity in children and adolescents: A meta-analysis. *Obes. Rev.* **2014**, *15*, 666–675. [CrossRef] [PubMed]
48. Sallis, J.; Prochaska, J.; Taylor, W. A review of correlates of physical activity. *Med. Sci. Sport. Exerc.* **2000**, *32*, 963–975. [CrossRef]
49. Pearson, N.; Biddle, S.J.H. Sedentary behavior and dietary intake in children, adolescents, and adults: A systematic review. *Am. J. Prev. Med.* **2011**, *41*, 178–188. [CrossRef] [PubMed]
50. Ottevaere, C.; Huybrechts, I.; Béghin, L.; Cuenca-Garcia, M.; de Bourdeaudhuij, I.; Gottrand, F.; Hagströmer, M.; Kafatos, A.; Le Donne, C.; Moreno, L.A.; et al. Relationship between self-reported dietary intake and physical activity levels among adolescents: The HELENA study. *Int. J. Behav. Nutr. Phys. Act.* **2011**, *8*, 8. [CrossRef] [PubMed]
51. Pereira, S.; Katzmarzyk, P.T.; Gomes, T.N.; Borges, A.; Santos, D.; Souza, M.; dos Santos, F.K.; Chaves, R.N.; Champagne, C.M.; Barreira, T.V.; et al. Profiling physical activity, diet, screen and sleep habits in Portuguese children. *Nutrients* **2015**, *7*, 4345–4362. [CrossRef] [PubMed]
52. Vissers, P.A.J.; Jones, A.P.; van Sluijs, E.M.F.; Jennings, A.; Welch, A.; Cassidy, A.; Griffin, S.J. Association between diet and physical activity and sedentary behaviours in 9–10-year-old British White children. *Public Health* **2012**, *127*, 231–240. *[CrossRef]* [PubMed]
53. Jago, R; Ness, A.R; Emment, P.; Mattocks, C.; Jones, L.; Riddoch, C.J. Obesogenic diet and physical activity behaviours: Independent or associated behaviours in adolescents. *Public Health Nutr.* **2010**, *13*, 673–681. [CrossRef] [PubMed]
54. Nelson, T.D.; Lundahl, A.; Molfese, D.L.; Waford, R.N.; Roman, A.; Gozal, D.; Molfese, V.J.; Ferguson, M.C. Estimating child sleep from parent report of time in bed: Development and evaluation of adjustment approaches. *J. Pediatr. Psychol.* **2014**, *39*, 624–632. [CrossRef] [PubMed]
55. Short, M.A.; Gradisar, M.; Lack, L.C.; Wright, H.R.; Chatburn, A. Estimating adolescent sleep patterns: Parent reports versus adolescent self-report surveys, sleep diaries, and actigraphy. *Nat. Sci. Sleep* **2013**, *5*, 23–26. [CrossRef] [PubMed]
56. Yamakita, M.; Sato, M.; Ando, D.; Suzuki, K.; Yamagata, Z. Availability of a simple self-report sleep questionnaire for 9- to 12-year-old children Study participants. *Sleep Biol. Rhythms* **2014**, *12*, 279–288. [CrossRef]
57. Ekstedt, M.; Nyberg, G.; Ingre, M.; Ekblom, Ö.; Marcus, C. Sleep, physical activity and BMI in six to ten-year-old children measured by accelerometry: A cross-sectional study. *Int. J. Behav. Nutr. Phys. Act.* **2013**, *10*, 1. [CrossRef] [PubMed]
58. Khan, M.K.A.; Chu, Y.L.; Kirk, S.F.L.; Veugelers, P.J. Are sleep duration and sleep quality associated with diet quality, physical activity, and body weight status? A population-based study of Canadian children. *Can. J. Public Health* **2015**, *106*, e277–e282. [CrossRef] [PubMed]
59. Jimenez-Pavon, D.; Kelly, J.; Reilly, J.J. Associations between objectively measured habitual physical activity and adiposity in children and adolescents: Systematic review. *Int. J. Pediatr. Obes.* **2010**, *5*, 3–18. [CrossRef] [PubMed]

60. Parikh, T.; Stratton, G. Influence of intensity of physical activity on adiposity and cardiorespiratory fitness in 518 year olds. *Sports Med.* **2011**, *41*, 477–488. [CrossRef] [PubMed]

61. Roman-Viñas, B.; Chaput, J.-P.; Katzmarzyk, P.T.; Fogelholm, M.; Lambert, E.V.; Maher, C.; Maia, J.; Olds, T.; Onywera, V.; Sarmiento, O.L.; et al. Proportion of children meeting recommendations for 24-hour movement guidelines and associations with adiposity in a 12-country study. *Int. J. Behav. Nutr. Phys. Act.* **2016**, *13*, 123. [CrossRef] [PubMed]

62. Kelly, B.; Halford, J.C.G.; Boyland, E.J.; Chapman, K.; Bautista-Castaño, I.; Berg, C.; Caroli, M.; Cook, B.; Coutinho, J.G.; Effertz, T.; et al. Television food advertising to children: A global perspective. *Am. J. Public Health* **2010**, *100*, 1730–1736. [CrossRef] [PubMed]

63. Boyland, E.J.; Halford, J.C.G. Television advertising and branding. Effects on eating behaviour and food preferences in children. *Appetite* **2013**, *62*, 236–241. [CrossRef] [PubMed]

64. Hysing, M.; Pallesen, S.; Stormark, K.M.; Jakobsen, R.; Lundervold, A.J.; Sivertsen, B. Sleep and use of electronic devices in adolescence: Results from a large population-based study. *BMJ Open* **2015**, *5*, e006748. [CrossRef] [PubMed]

65. Marques, A.; Ekelund, U.; Sardinha, L.B. Associations between organized sports participation and objectively measured physical activity, sedentary time and weight status in youth. *J. Sci. Med. Sport* **2015**, *19*, 1–4. [CrossRef] [PubMed]

66. Morgan, K.; Hallingberg, B.; Littlecott, H.; Murphy, S.; Fletcher, A.; Roberts, C.; Moore, G. Predictors of physical activity and sedentary behaviours among 11-16 year olds: Multilevel analysis of the 2013 Health Behaviour in School-aged Children (HBSC) study in Wales. *BMC Public Health* **2016**, *16*, 569. [CrossRef] [PubMed]

67. Hatch, K.E. Determining the Effects of Technology on Children. 2011. Available online: http://digitalcommons.uri.edu/srhonorsprog/260/ (access on 14 February 2018).

68. Gorely, T.; Biddle, S.; Marshall, S.; Cameron, N.; Cassey, N. The association between distance to school, physical activity and sedentary behaviors in adolescents: Project STIL. *Pediatr. Exerc. Sci.* **2009**, *21*, 450–461. [CrossRef] [PubMed]

69. Arundell, L.; Hinkley, T.; Veitch, J.; Salmon, J. Contribution of the after-school period to children's daily participation in physical activity and sedentary behaviours. *PLoS ONE* **2015**, *10*, 1–11. [CrossRef] [PubMed]

70. Ar-Yuwat, S.; Clark, M.J.; Hunter, A.; James, K.S. Determinants of physical activity in primary school students using the health belief model. *J. Multidiscip. Healthc.* **2013**, *6*, 119–126. [CrossRef] [PubMed]

71. Feldman, D.E.; Barnett, T.; Shrier, I.; Rossignol, M.; Abenhaim, L. Is physical activity differentially associated with different types of sedentary pursuits? *Arch. Pediatr. Adolesc. Med.* **2003**, *157*, 797–802. [CrossRef] [PubMed]

72. Jago, R.; Sebire, S.J.; Gorely, T.; Cillero, I.H.; Biddle, S.J.H. " I'm on it 24/7 at the moment ": A qualitative examination of multi-screen viewing behaviours among UK 10-11 year olds. *Int. J. Behav. Nutr. Phys. Act.* **2011**, 1–8. [CrossRef] [PubMed]

73. Pate, R.R.; Taverno Ross, S.E.; Liese, A.D.; Dowda, M. Associations among physical activity, diet quality, and weight status in US adults. *Med. Sci. Sports Exerc.* **2015**, *47*, 743–750. [CrossRef] [PubMed]

74. Fortes, L.; Morgado, F.; Almeida, S.; Ferreira, M. Eating behavior and physical activity in adolescents. *Rev. Nutr.* **2013**, *26*, 529–537. [CrossRef]

75. Atkin, A.J.; Gorely, T.; Clemes, S.A.; Yates, T.; Edwardson, C.; Brage, S.; Salmon, J.; Marshall, S.J.; Biddle, S.J.H. Methods of measurement in epidemiology: Sedentary behaviour. *Int. J. Epidemiol.* **2012**, *41*, 1460–1471. [CrossRef] [PubMed]

76. Hjorth, M.F.; Chaput, J.P.; Damsgaard, C.T.; Dalskov, S.M.; Andersen, R.; Astrup, A.; Michaelsen, K.F.; Tetens, I.; Ritz, C.; Sjödin, A. Low physical activity level and short sleep duration are associated with an increased cardio-metabolic risk profile: A longitudinal study in 8–11 year old Danish children. *PLoS ONE* **2014**, *9*. [CrossRef] [PubMed]

77. Wang, L.; Luo, J.; Luo, J.; Gao, W.; Kong, J. The effect of Internet use on adolescents' lifestyles: A national survey. *Comput. Human Behav.* **2012**, *28*, 2007–2013. [CrossRef]

78. Gordon-Larsen, P.; Adair, L.S.; Popkin, B.M. Ethnic differences in physical activity and inactivity patterns and overweight status. *Obes. Res.* **2002**, *10*, 141–149. [CrossRef] [PubMed]

79. Elsenburg, L.K.; Corpeleijn, E.; van Sluijs, E.M.F.; Atkin, A.J. Clustering and correlates of multiple health behaviours in 9–10 year old children. *PLoS ONE* **2014**, *9*, e99498. [CrossRef] [PubMed]
80. Maitland, C.; Stratton, G.; Foster, S.; Braham, R.; Rosenberg, M. A place for play? The influence of the home physical environment on children' s physical activity and sedentary behaviour. *Int. J. Behav. Nutr. Phys. Act.* **2013**, *10*, 1. [CrossRef] [PubMed]

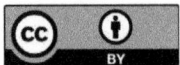

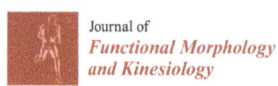

Journal of
Functional Morphology and Kinesiology

Article

Physical Fitness Evaluation of School Children in Southern Italy: A Cross Sectional Evaluation

Ewan Thomas * and Antonio Palma

Sport and Exercise Sciences Research Unit, University of Palermo, 90146 Palermo, Italy; antonio.palma@unipa.it
* Correspondence: ewan.thomas@unipa.it; Tel.: +39-320-889-9934

Received: 20 December 2017; Accepted: 14 February 2018; Published: 26 February 2018

Abstract: The aim of this work was to evaluate the fitness levels of different physical components in schoolchildren in southern Italy and identify age-related effects of physical performance. One hundred and fifty-four schoolchildren with ages ranging between 6 and 10 years (age 8.1 ± 1.45 years; 33.70 ± 10.25 kg; 131.50 ± 13.60 cm) were recruited for the investigation. Each scholar underwent a fitness-test battery composed of five elements. A Hand-Grip Strength Test to assess the strength of the hand muscles, a Standing Broad Jump Test to assess lower body explosive strength, a Sit-Up Test to exhaustion to evaluate abdominal muscular endurance, a 4×10-m Shuttle Run Test to assess agility, and a 20-m sprint test to assess speed. Cross-sectional analysis revealed that boys perform better than girls and that age affects performance. Lower limb measures show a significant increase after 8 years of age, whereas upper limb measures show a significant increase at 7 and 10 years of age. No age-related differences were found in muscular endurance measures. It is possible to consider age-related performance measures to program exercise interventions that follow the growth characteristics of schoolchildren.

Keywords: physical fitness; assessment; children; evaluation

1. Introduction

Physical activity (PA) is a key component in order to maintain and improve health, including physical, mental, and emotional health [1–4]. A considerable amount of evidence exists that supports the concept that PA is able to improve musculoskeletal health, improve cardiovascular fitness, and improve body composition and overall physical fitness [5]. The latter is defined as a state of wellbeing, which refers to the ability to perform daily tasks, sports, or occupations without undue fatigue [6].

Fitness tests are usually assessed in laboratories or fields. However, laboratory tests are more costly and time consuming. Notwithstanding field tests are in general less accurate, are widely used for their lower costs, and require less time for their administration [7].

In order to assess physical fitness through field-based fitness tests, different attempts have been made in both children and adolescents. Successful examples are the Assessing Levels of Physical Activity study (ALPHA study) [8], which aimed to identify reliable fitness tests for children and adolescents; the AVENA study, which aimed to evaluate cardiovascular fitness in youth around Europe [9]; the Healthy Lifestyle in Europe by Nutrition in Adolescence study (the HELENA study) [10], which evaluated physical fitness over 10 European nations; FitnessGram [11], whose purpose was to increase the levels of physical activity in children in the United States; and EUROFIT [12], a program in Europe. All these attempts firstly detected the reliability of the fitness tests for specific populations and secondly provided age-related fitness percentile values [13,14].

In a previous study, we identified five field-based fitness tests to evaluate the level of physical fitness in adolescents and subsequently, in a second study, evaluated physical fitness of adolescents using the selected fitness tests in the context of the Adolescents Surveillance System and Obesity prevention study (ASSO project) [6,15]. These were chosen according to their feasibility, safeness, reliability, and low cost. These tests were the standing broad jump for the evaluation of lower limb strength, the hand-grip test for the evaluation of the strength of the upper limbs, the sit-up to exhaustion for the evaluation of abdominal muscular endurance, the 4 × 10-m shuttle run for the evaluation of agility, and the 20-m shuttle run test for the evaluation of aerobic capacity. Notwithstanding that such a fitness battery was used in adolescents, other studies such as AVENA, FitnessGram, or EUROFIT, have used similar fitness batteries to evaluate physical fitness levels in children [11,12,16,17]. Another similar battery is that proposed by the PREFIT study used in Spanish schoolchildren [18].

In schools or sports, children are generally classified in age groups, and this grouping is usually done according to the age of birth, thus a one year difference will be often present [19]. During development, older individuals usually perform better [20], defining what is known as the relative age effect [21]. If such an effect was not relevant, then it would be of no use to group children according to their age. The age-related effect may be applicable to both physical and mental aspects. To the best of our knowledge, age thresholds at which physical development may induce significant variations in physical fitness has not received considerable attention, thus, the aim of this study was twofold: firstly, to evaluate the fitness levels in schoolchildren from southern Italy through a validated field-based fitness battery and secondly, to determine whether age-related effects in physical performance for each selected measure is present.

2. Materials and Methods

2.1. Participants

One hundred and fifty-four school children with ages ranging between 6 and 10 years (age 8.1 ± 1.45 years; 33.7 ± 10.25 kg; 131.5 ± 13.6 cm) from an elementary school in southern Italy were recruited for this investigation. The school was selected within the context of a project (Alfabetizzazione Motoria) to which the school had adhered that was organized by the National Olympic Committee (CONI) and by the Ministry of Education of the University and Research (MIUR) with the aim to promote physical activity in elementary schools. All schoolchildren were tested at the beginning of the project. An initial number of 169 children had been tested, however, only the children that performed all the selected tests of the fitness battery were included for the analysis. Children with medical issues or physical and mental disabilities were not included in the study. The final 154 participants were 80 males (age 8.10 ± 1.40 years; 34.70 ± 9.90 kg; 132.90 ± 8.30 cm) and 74 females (age 8 ± 1.50 years; 32.70 ± 10.60 kg; 129.70 ± 17.70 cm). The principles of the Italian data protection (196/2003) were guaranteed. The Ethical Committee of the DISMOT department approved the project (approval number: 4, approval date: 29 July 2010). The study was undertaken in accordance with the deontological norms laid down in the Helsinki Declaration and the European Union recommendations for Good Clinical Practice.

2.2. Methods

The participants undertook a modified ASSO Fitness Test Battery (FTB) [6] that comprised of five selected tests for the assessment of the physical fitness components: (1) the Hand-Grip Strength Test (HG) to assess upper body strength, (2) the Standing Broad Jump Test (SBJ) to assess lower body explosive strength, (3) the Sit-Up Test to exhaustion (SUT) to assess abdominal muscular endurance, (4) the 4 × 10-m Shuttle Run Test (4 × 10 mSRT) to assess agility, and (5) the 20-m sprint test (20 mST) to assess speed [6,16,22,23]. All tests were performed three times and the best score was retained for investigation except for the sit-up test to exhaustion, which was performed only once. At least one parent of each participant had to present a signed consent form in order to allow the children to participate in the study.

All participants were tested during school hours, from 9 to 12 am, by the same investigator. One test per day was administered, in order to allow each child to properly understand the indications of the investigator and not bias the results through progressive fatiguing.

Prior to the administration of the fitness battery, anthropometric measures of each participant were assessed using a scale with a 0.1 kg sensitivity (Seca 709, Seca, Hamburg, Germany) for weight and a wall-stadiometer with a 1 mm sensitivity (Seca 220, Seca) for height.

On the first day, the HG was administered. The test consisted of grabbing a digital handheld dynamometer (KERN MAP 80 K1, Kern & Sohn GmbH, Balingen, Germany) with the arm fully extended, not touching the body, and squeezing the dynamometer at maximum strength. This task was carried out while standing. Each participant repeated the task three times with the right hand (HG R) and three times with the left hand (HG L). Between each task each participant had a two-minute rest to allow for a full recovery. The highest of the three trials was considered for statistical analysis.

On the second day, the participants had to perform the SBJ. The test consisted of jumping forward the maximum possible distance, starting from a standing position. Each participant was required to stand with his/her heels on a line that represented the starting point. The feet had to be parallel to each other. Each participant was allowed to squat before the jump and swing the arms forward during the jump. The measurement of the SBJ was calculated from the starting line to the point at which the heels of the participant touched the ground. A tape measure was used to evaluate performance. Each participant performed three trials with a two-minute rest between each task and the greatest of the three tasks was considered for analysis.

On the third day, the participants performed the SUT. The participants had to lay supine on the floor with the knee joints flexed at 90°, hands at the side of their head, and their elbows pointing straight forward. The correct sit-up execution was considered when the elbows touched the knees during the concentric phase of the movement and then the shoulders touched the floor during the eccentric phase of the movement [22]. If the participants were not able to lift the back from the floor a number of 0 repetitions were counted. The test ended when the participants were not able to perform the repetitions with the correct form above described. The participants were not allowed to recover during the test. The SUT was performed only once.

On the fourth day, the participants were asked to perform the 4 × 10 mSRT. Each participant was asked to run back and forth four times within two lines 10 m apart at his/her maximum possible speed. Each participant had to start behind the start line and had to cross the opposite line before they had to change direction and start running to the opposite line again. Each participant started running upon receiving the verbal command "go" from the investigator. The test ended when the participant crossed the finish line at the end of the fourth shuttle. Time was measured with a stopwatch. Each participant performed three tasks with a two-minute rest between each task. The fastest of the three measures was retained for investigation.

On the fifth day, the participants were asked to perform a 20 mST. Each participant was asked to run within two lines 20 m apart at the maximum possible speed. Each participant had to start behind the start line. The test started when each participated received the verbal command "go" from the investigator and ended when the participant crossed the finish line. Time was measured with a stopwatch. Each participant performed three tasks with a two-minute rest between each task. The fastest of the three measures was retained for investigation.

2.3. Statistical Analysis

Descriptive statistics were used for anthropometric parameters and for performance representation of the entire sample and the stratified samples. Unpaired *t*-tests with Welch's correction were used to evaluate differences between performance measures and between age groups of the same performance measure. ANOVA was used to determine a significant effect of age on performance and a subsequent intra-group analysis to identify the age thresholds. Analysis was performed using SPSS Statistica 10.0

(Statsoft, Tulsa, OK, USA) for Windows and Prism 6 (GraphPad software, Inc., La Jolla, CA, USA) for graph creation.

3. Results

Descriptive characteristics of the sample are presented in Table 1.

Table 1. Descriptive characteristics of the sample.

	Male					
Age (years)	8.10 ± 1.40	6	7	8	9	10
Subjects (n)	80	14	13	19	17	17
Body Mass (kg)	34.70 ± 9.90	26.1 ± 6.3	30.6 ± 7.6	33.9 ± 9.6	38.6 ± 9.6	42.2 ± 8.0
Height (cm)	132.90 ± 8.30	123.1 ± 6.1	127.5 ± 6.0	133.4 ± 5.8	137.0 ± 6.5	140.8 ± 4.1
	Female					
Age (years)	8 ± 1.50	6	7	8	9	10
Subjects (n)	74	17	17	8	15	17
Body Mass (kg)	32.70 ± 10.60	25.1 ± 4.8	28.5 ± 6.2	31.6 ± 9.5	39.4 ± 11.8	38.2 ± 11.0
Height (cm)	129.70 ± 17.70	119.2 ± 4.8	118.7 ± 28.3	131.0 ± 4.3	138.2 ± 6.7	142.8 ± 7.0

Data are presented as means ± standard deviations.

The general outcome of the performance measures shows an increase according to age in both males and females. This trend is evident in all physical measures, as shown in Table 2. Stratified performance measures are reported in Table 3 for male participants and Table 4 for female participants. Single performance measures for both males and females are shown in Figures 1–5.

Table 2. Performance measures of the entire sample.

Age	SBJ (cm)	4 × 10 m (s)	SUT (reps)	HG R (kg)	HG L (kg)	20 mST (s)
6	115.6 ± 16.9	15.8 ± 1.6	16.7 ± 16.6	7.7 ± 2.2	7.2 ± 2.1	5.49 ± 0.52
7	118.3 ± 17.4	15.6 ± 1.7	24.9 ± 21.9	10.6 ± 2.4	9.8 ± 2.5	5.15 ± 0.59
8	126.9 ± 18.8	14.3 ± 1.9	42.4 ± 41.3	13.1 ± 3.2	11.2 ± 3.2	5.09 ± 0.62
9	137.6 ± 19.1	14.5 ± 1.5	50.3 ± 46.2	14.7 ± 3.4	13.2 ± 3.6	4.98 ± 0.60
10	140.6 ± 18.3	13.4 ± 1.1	55.91 ± 34.9	16.5 ± 3.3	14.7 ± 3.5	4.78 ± 0.42

Data are presented as means ± standard deviations. SBJ: Standing Broad Jump Test; SUT: Sit-Up Test to exhaustion; HG R: Hand-Grip Strength Test for the right hand; HG L: Hand-Grip Strength Test for the left hand; 20 mST: 20-m sprint test.

Table 3. Performance measures of the male participants.

Age	SBJ (cm)	4 × 10 m (s)	SUT (reps)	HG R (kg)	HG L (kg)	20 mST (s)
6	122.1 ± 16.8	15.4 ± 1.95	11.2 ± 8.9	8.4 ± 2.3	7.7 ± 2.3	5.36 ± 0.55
7	124.8 ± 20.2	15.8 ± 1.87	25.85 ± 28.9	11.8 ± 2.2	10.7 ± 2.9	5.01 ± 0.56
8	135.5 ± 18.4	13.6 ± 1.2	47.0 ± 46.7	13.6 ± 3.2	11.9 ± 3.4	5.08 ± 0.71
9	142.1 ± 19.1	13.8 ± 1.5	68.1 ± 54.9	15.5 ± 3.8	14.2 ± 3.9	4.77 ± 0.55
10	143.4 ± 15.5	12.9 ± 0.8	64.1 ± 32.5	18.4 ± 3.3	16.2 ± 3.6	4.62 ± 0.30

Data are presented as means ± standard deviations.

Table 4. Performance measures of the female participants.

Age	SBJ (cm)	4 × 10 m (s)	SUT (reps)	HG R (kg)	HG L (kg)	20 mST (s)
6	110.3 ± 14.6	16.1 ± 1.2	21.3 ± 20.1	7.1 ± 1.5	6.8 ± 0.9	5.59 ± 0.48
7	113.3 ± 13.6	16.1 ± 1.4	24.2 ± 15.5	9.7 ± 2.1	9.1 ± 1.9	5.26 ± 0.61
8	118.2 ± 15.3	15.8 ± 2.4	30.9 ± 21.4	11.6 ± 2.9	9.71 ± 2.1	5.11 ± 0.35
9	126.5 ± 14.4	15.1 ± 1.2	32.7 ± 26.8	13.9 ± 2.9	12.2 ± 3.2	5.18 ± 0.60
10	137.9 ± 18.2	13.9 ± 1.2	48.2 ± 36.2	14.8 ± 2.2	13.3 ± 2.8	4.92 ± 0.47

Data are presented as means ± standard deviations.

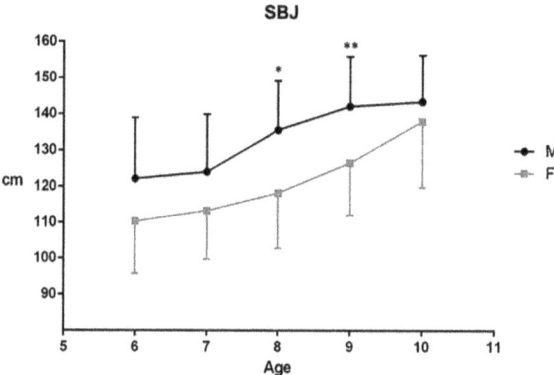

Figure 1. Standing broad jump of male and female schoolchildren stratified by age. Differences between male (M) and female (F) * $p < 0.05$; ** $p < 0.01$.

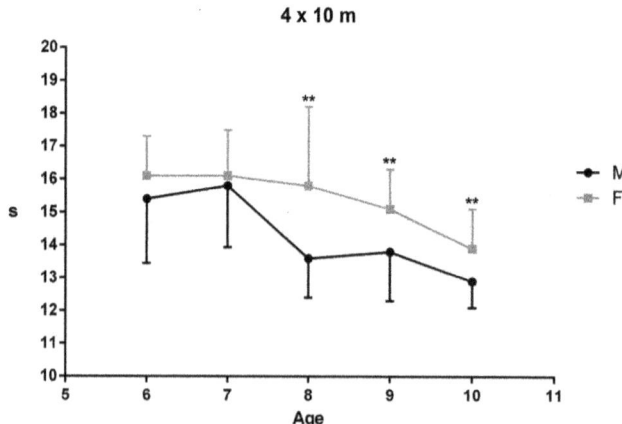

Figure 2. 4 × 10 m shuttle run test of male and female schoolchildren stratified by age. Differences between male (M) and female (F) ** $p < 0.01$.

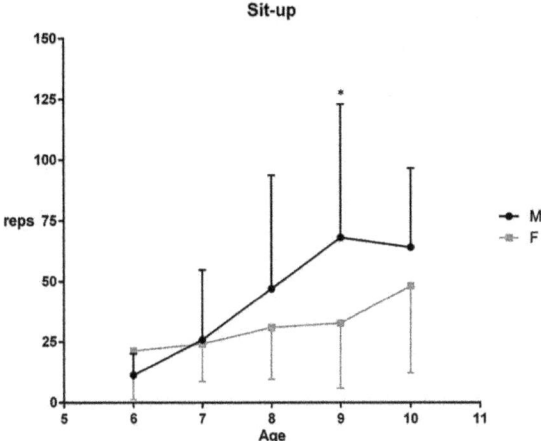

Figure 3. Sit-up test of male and female schoolchildren stratified by age. Differences between male (M) and female (F) * $p < 0.05$.

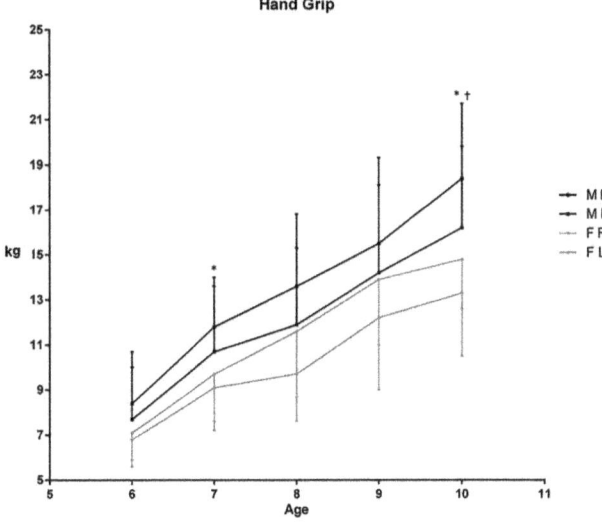

Figure 4. Hand-grip test results for both the right (R) and left (L) hands of male (M) and female (F) schoolchildren stratified by age. Differences between male and female * $p < 0.05$; † $p < 0.001$.

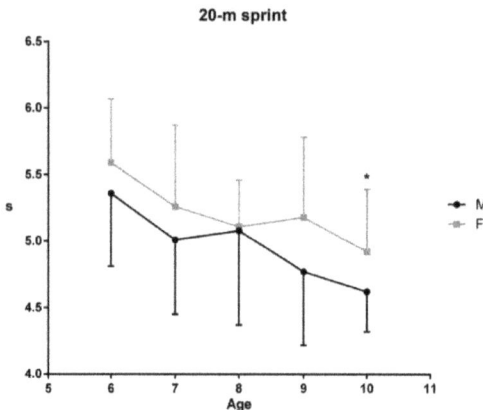

Figure 5. 20-m sprint test of male and female schoolchildren stratified by age. Differences between male (M) and female (F). * $p < 0.05$.

Statistical analysis showed significant differences between male and female participants across all tests, with better performance measures for the male schoolchildren. Analysis of variance has also shown a significant effect of age on the performance measures. However, when sub-analysis on single components was performed to determine which age groups had the greatest differences, each test showed different outcomes. In particular, a significant effect on the 4 × 10 mSRT was evident between 6 and 7 years of age, and in the HG between 7 and 8 years of age. This analysis, however, did not take into account gender differences. Major results are presented in Table 5.

Table 5. Statistical differences between groups.

Tests	Gender	Age	6	7	8	9	10
SBJ	<0.0001	<0.0001	ns	ns	0.047	0.007	ns
4 × 10 m	<0.0001	<0.0001 [b]	ns	ns	0.004	0.008	0.005
SUT	0.022	<0.0001	ns	ns	ns	0.03	ns
HG R	0.0002	<0.0001 [a,b]	ns	0.011	ns	ns	0.0005
HG L	0.0012	<0.0001 [a]	ns	0.048	ns	ns	0.012
20 mST	0.0047	<0.0001	ns	ns	ns	ns	0.034

Gender: unpaired *t*-test between male and female of the whole sample; Age: one-way ANOVA [a]: 6 vs. 7, [b]: 7 vs. 8, between age groups regardless of gender; Age groups (6, 7, 8, 9, 10) unpaired *t*-test between male and female of the same age; ns: not significant.

At 7 and 10 years of age the strength of the upper limbs shows significant differences between male and female participants, whereas the lower limbs (SBJ) show differences in performance only between 8 and 9 years of age across gender. A significant difference between male and female schoolchildren is also shown at ages 8, 9, and 10 in regard to the 4 × 10-m shuttle run test used for agility.

4. Discussion

The aims of this study were twofold: (1) to assess physical fitness in schoolchildren and (2) to identify the age-related effects on physical fitness in this population. Physical fitness increases according to age, thus there is a significant age-related effect for all physical measures. Secondly, there is a significant difference between male and female schoolchildren, with the male children performing significantly better than the female children. In addition, age thresholds of increased performance have been determined and a significant increase of the strength of the lower limbs is present at 8 years of age, whereas a significant increase of the strength of the upper limbs is present at 7 and 10 years of age. The speed and agility measures are seen to significantly increase from 9 to 10 years of age.

The increase of performance according to age and the differences between male and female schoolchildren are in line with other studies in the literature [24–26]. In a sample of German schoolchildren [24], a significant age effect was seen amongst different fitness tests. In particular, an increase of the upper limb strength measures was seen in both boys and girls around 9 and 10 years of age. Another population study based on Spanish schoolchildren evaluated the physical fitness of 1725 children with ages ranging from 6 to 12 years, using the FitnessGram battery. The results of the study posit increased physical fitness of boys compared to girls in all fitness measures, showing a linear increase across age [25]. It is interesting to note that our modified ASSO FTB shares common fitness tests with the FitnessGram battery (Hand-grip, Standing Broad jump Test, Sit-up test, and a shuttle run test) and that our physical measures are in agreement with those of Gulias-Gonzales et al. [25]. A third study analyzing Polish schoolchildren [26] used the EUROFIT battery to assess physical fitness in children and adolescents. The results provide percentile values over a large population for 14 different fitness measures, of which three are in common with our battery (Hand-grip, standing broad jump, and the 4 × 10-m shuttle run). Notwithstanding the analyzed population comes from a different geographical area, the results support the greater physical fitness of boys compared to girls, increased measures according to age, and similar physical outcomes when compared to our analyzed sample from southern Italy.

Many studies have provided percentile values for physical fitness tests for both children and adolescents and the results of all these studies are again in agreement with our results, with boys performing better than girls, and older children performing better than younger ones [24]. All these studies, in particular, have observed increased performance values for strength (e.g., Hand-grip), power (e.g., standing broad jump), agility (e.g., 4 × 10-m shuttle run), muscular endurance (e.g., Sit-ups), and endurance (e.g., 20 m shuttle run test) [27,28]. The reported tests are all included in our ASSO FTB, except for the endurance measures. These outcomes are helpful to consider for the identification of physical fitness characteristics in a specific sample of schoolchildren, and the results obtained here seem similar to other cohorts analyzed elsewhere.

The progressive stages of puberty, revised by Schell et al. [29], highlight an s-shaped development from birth to adulthood, with a fast growth from 0 to 6 years old, followed by a constant growth from 7 to 11 years old, and fast growth again during puberty. Genes, hormones, nutrients, environment, and physiological systems such as the genital system influence this growth pattern. The most evident change may be seen in anthropometric characteristics such as weight and height that will influence the athletic performance with changes in energy expenditure, as well as force and power production [30].

The review by Ford et al. [30] tried to determine critical periods during development to identify performance changes, and several aspects have been taken into account. In regard to muscle growth, it has been seen that at 7 years of age in both males and females there is a significant increase of muscle mass, especially in the cross-sectional area. Concomitantly, between 6 and 8 years of age a remodeling of the cerebral cortex and increase of the dendritic density is also present. This developmental stage may explain why between 7 and 8 years of age a significant increase in the performance of the upper and lower limbs is displayed. Between 8 and 10 years of age, the most prevalent developmental increases are seen on the hormonal system and in the aerobic capacity [22]. Around 9 years of age, there is an increased release of catecholamines and a higher response to insulin and glucagon, whereas development of the cardiorespiratory system is prevalent around 10 years of age. Between 10 and 12 years of age there is notable development of nerve pathways and increases in motor skill development are also present [22]. These developmental stages are useful to explain our results, where the running skills of the children start to increase at 10 years of age. The main limit of our study is the sample size, which in our case is confined to only one elementary school. Thus, this means that the results may be relevant to the analyzed sample

J. Funct. Morphol. Kinesiol. **2018**, *3*, 14

and not extended for general conclusions. Notwithstanding such limits, the results of this study seem to be in line with other studies in the literature.

5. Conclusions

An age relative effect is present between 6 and 10 years of age with differences between the analyzed male and female schoolchildren from southern Italy. Our results highlight that the strength of the upper limbs develops earlier than lower limbs and that speed and agility are greater around 10 years of age.

The results of the present study support the already existing literature and could help teachers and sport professionals to understand the different fitness developmental phases through the use of the selected fitness tests and motor development intervention programs.

Author Contributions: Ewan Thomas has conceived the manuscript, collected and analyzed the data and drafted the manuscript. Antonio Palma has revised the drafted manuscript and gave the final approval.

Conflicts of Interest: The authors declare that they have no conflict of interest.

References

1. Ortega, F.B.; Ruiz, J.R.; Castillo, M.J.; Moreno, L.A.; Urzanqui, A.; Gonzalez-Gross, M.; Sjostrom, M.; Gutierrez, A.; Group, A.S. Health-related physical fitness according to chronological and biological age in adolescents. The AVENA study. *J. Sports Med. Phys. Fit.* **2008**, *48*, 371–379.
2. Eime, R.M.; Young, J.A.; Harvey, J.T.; Charity, M.J.; Payne, W.R. A systematic review of the psychological and social benefits of participation in sport for children and adolescents: Informing development of a conceptual model of health through sport. *Int. J. Behav. Nutr. Phys. Act.* **2013**, *10*, 98. [CrossRef] [PubMed]
3. Hajek, P.; Stead, L. F. *Global Recommendations on Physical Activity for Health*; WHO Press: Geneva, Switzerland, 2010.
4. Paoli, A.; Bianco, A. Not all exercises are created equal. *Am. J. Cardiol.* **2012**, *109*, 305. [CrossRef] [PubMed]
5. Ortega, F.B.; Ruiz, J.R.; Castillo, M.J.; Sjostrom, M. Physical fitness in childhood and adolescence: A powerful marker of health. *Int. J. Obes.* **2008**, *32*, 1–11. [CrossRef] [PubMed]
6. Bianco, A.; Jemni, M.; Thomas, E.; Patti, A.; Paoli, A.; Ramos Roque, J.; Palma, A.; Mammina, C.; Tabacchi, G. A systematic review to determine reliability and usefulness of the field-based test batteries for the assessment of physical fitness in adolescents—The ASSO Project. *Int. J. Occup. Med. Environ. Health* **2015**, *28*, 445–478. [CrossRef] [PubMed]
7. Heyward, V.H.; Gibson, A. *Advanced Fitness Assessment and Exercise Prescription 7th Edition*; Human Kinetics: Champagne, IL, USA, 2014.
8. Ruiz, J.R.; Castro-Pinero, J.; Espana-Romero, V.; Artero, E.G.; Ortega, F.B.; Cuenca, M.M.; Jimenez-Pavon, D.; Chillon, P.; Girela-Rejon, M.J.; Mora, J.; et al. Field-based fitness assessment in young people: The ALPHA health-related fitness test battery for children and adolescents. *Br. J. Sports Med.* **2011**, *45*, 518–524. [CrossRef] [PubMed]
9. Ortega, F.B.; Ruiz, J.R.; Castillo, M.J.; Moreno, L.A.; Gonzalez-Gross, M.; Warnberg, J.; Gutierrez, A.; Group, A. Low level of physical fitness in Spanish adolescents. Relevance for future cardiovascular health (Avena study). *Rev. Esp. Cardiol.* **2005**, *58*, 898–909. [CrossRef] [PubMed]
10. Ortega, F.B.; Artero, E.G.; Ruiz, J.R.; Vicente-Rodriguez, G.; Bergman, P.; Hagstromer, M.; Ottevaere, C.; Nagy, E.; Konsta, O.; Rey-Lopez, J.P.; et al. Reliability of health-related physical fitness tests in European adolescents. The HELENA Study. *Int. J. Obes.* **2008**, *32*, S49–57. [CrossRef] [PubMed]
11. Morrow, J.R., Jr.; Martin, S.B.; Jackson, A.W. Reliability and validity of the FITNESSGRAM: Quality of teacher-collected health-related fitness surveillance data. *Res. Q. Exerc. Sport* **2010**, *81*, S24–30. [CrossRef] [PubMed]
12. Tomkinson, G.R.; Carver, K.D.; Atkinson, F.; Daniell, N.D.; Lewis, L.K.; Fitzgerald, J.S.; Lang, J.J.; Ortega, F.B. European normative values for physical fitness in children and adolescents aged 9–17 years: Results from 2,779,165 Eurofit performances representing 30 countries. *Br. J. Sports Med.* **2017**. [CrossRef] [PubMed]
13. Ortega, F.B.; Artero, E.G.; Ruiz, J.R.; Espana-Romero, V.; Jimenez-Pavon, D.; Vicente-Rodriguez, G.; Moreno, L.A.; Manios, Y.; Beghin, L.; Ottevaere, C.; et al. Physical fitness levels among European adolescents: The HELENA study. *Br. J. Sports Med.* **2011**, *45*, 20–29. [CrossRef] [PubMed]

14. Vanhelst, J.; Beghin, L.; Fardy, P.S.; Ulmer, Z.; Czaplicki, G. Reliability of health-related physical fitness tests in adolescents: The MOVE Program. *Clin. Physiol. Funct. Imaging* **2016**, *36*, 106–111. [CrossRef] [PubMed]

15. Bianco, A.; Mammina, C.; Jemni, M.; Filippi, A.R.; Patti, A.; Thomas, E.; Paoli, A.; Palma, A.; Tabacchi, G. A Fitness Index model for Italian adolescents living in Southern Italy: The ASSO project. *J. Sports Med. Phys. Fit.* **2016**, *56*, 1279–1288.

16. Artero, E.G.; Espana-Romero, V.; Castro-Pinero, J.; Ortega, F.B.; Suni, J.; Castillo-Garzon, M.J.; Ruiz, J.R. Reliability of field-based fitness tests in youth. *Int. J. Sports Med.* **2011**, *32*, 159–169. [CrossRef] [PubMed]

17. Castro-Pinero, J.; Artero, E.G.; Espana-Romero, V.; Ortega, F.B.; Sjostrom, M.; Suni, J.; Ruiz, J.R. Criterion-related validity of field-based fitness tests in youth: A systematic review. *Br. J. Sports Med.* **2010**, *44*, 934–943. [CrossRef] [PubMed]

18. Ortega, F.B.; Cadenas-Sanchez, C.; Sanchez-Delgado, G.; Mora-Gonzalez, J.; Martinez-Tellez, B.; Artero, E.G.; Castro-Pinero, J.; Labayen, I.; Chillon, P.; Lof, M.; et al. Systematic review and proposal of a field-based physical fitness-test battery in preschool children: The PREFIT battery. *Sports Med.* **2015**, *45*, 533–555. [CrossRef] [PubMed]

19. Veldhuizen, S.; Cairney, J.; Hay, J.; Faught, B. Relative age effects in fitness testing in a general school sample: How relative are they? *J. Sports Sci.* **2015**, *33*, 109–115. [CrossRef] [PubMed]

20. Cobley, S.; Baker, J.; Wattie, N.; McKenna, J. Annual age-grouping and athlete development: A meta-analytical review of relative age effects in sport. *Sports Med.* **2009**, *39*, 235–256. [CrossRef] [PubMed]

21. Wattie, N.; Cobley, S.; Baker, J. Towards a unified understanding of relative age effects. *J. Sports Sci.* **2008**, *26*, 1403–1409. [CrossRef] [PubMed]

22. Bianco, A.; Lupo, C.; Alesi, M.; Spina, S.; Raccuglia, M.; Thomas, E.; Paoli, A.; Palma, A. The sit up test to exhaustion as a test for muscular endurance evaluation. *Springerplus* **2015**, *4*, 309. [CrossRef] [PubMed]

23. Ruiz, J.R.; Espana Romero, V.; Castro Pinero, J.; Artero, E.G.; Ortega, F.B.; Cuenca Garcia, M.; Jimenez Pavon, D.; Chillon, P.; Girela Rejon, M.J.; Mora, J.; et al. ALPHA-fitness test battery: Health-related field-based fitness tests assessment in children and adolescents. *Nutr. Hosp.* **2011**, *26*, 1210–1214. [PubMed]

24. Golle, K.; Muehlbauer, T.; Wick, D.; Granacher, U. Physical Fitness Percentiles of German Children Aged 9–12 Years: Findings from a Longitudinal Study. *PLoS ONE* **2015**, *10*, e0142393. [CrossRef] [PubMed]

25. Gulias-Gonzalez, R.; Sanchez-Lopez, M.; Olivas-Bravo, A.; Solera-Martinez, M.; Martinez-Vizcaino, V. Physical fitness in Spanish schoolchildren aged 6–12 years: Reference values of the battery EUROFIT and associated cardiovascular risk. *J. Sch. Health* **2014**, *84*, 625–635. [CrossRef] [PubMed]

26. Dobosz, J.; Mayorga-Vega, D.; Viciana, J. Percentile Values of Physical Fitness Levels among Polish Children Aged 7 to 19 Years—A Population-Based Study. *Cent. Eur. J. Public Health* **2015**, *23*, 340–351. [CrossRef] [PubMed]

27. Roriz De Oliveira, M.S.; Seabra, A.; Freitas, D.; Eisenmann, J.C.; Maia, J. Physical fitness percentile charts for children aged 6–10 from Portugal. *Sports Med. Phys. Fit.* **2014**, *54*, 780–792.

28. Castro-Pinero, J.; Gonzalez-Montesinos, J.L.; Mora, J.; Keating, X.D.; Girela-Rejon, M.J.; Sjostrom, M.; Ruiz, J.R. Percentile values for muscular strength field tests in children aged 6 to 17 years: Influence of weight status. *J. Strength Cond. Res.* **2009**, *23*, 2295–2310. [CrossRef] [PubMed]

29. Schell, L.M. Fetus into man: Physical growth from conception to maturity (revised and enlarged edition). *Am. J. Hum. Biol.* **1991**, *3*, 217–218. [CrossRef]

30. Ford, P.; Collins, D.; Bailey, R.; MacNamara, Á.; Pearce, G.; Toms, M. Participant development in sport and physical activity: The impact of biological maturation. *Eur. J. Sport Sci.* **2012**, *12*, 515–526. [CrossRef]

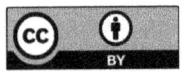

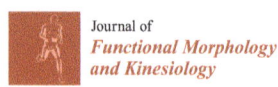

Journal of
Functional Morphology
and Kinesiology

Article

Do Young Elite Football Athletes Have the Same Strength and Power Characteristics as Senior Athletes?

Francisco Tavares [1,2], Bruno Mendes [3,4], Matthew Driller [1] and Sandro Freitas [3,4,*]

1   Faculty of Health, Sport and Human Performance, University of Waikato, Hamilton 3240, New Zealand;
     tavaresxico@gmail.com (F.T.); mdriller@waikato.ac.nz (M.D.)
2   Glasgow Warriors, Glasgow, UK
3   Benfica Lab, Lisbon 1500-313, Portugal; bmendes@slbenfica.pt
4   Faculty of Human Kinetics, University of Lisbon, Lisbon 1499-002, Portugal
*   Correspondence: sfreitas@fmh.ulisboa.pt; Tel.: +351-21-414-91-00

Received: 2 December 2017; Accepted: 12 December 2017; Published: 19 December 2017

Abstract: An increasing number of young football athletes are competing in elite senior level competitions. However, comparison of strength, power, and speed characteristics between young elite football athletes and their senior counterparts, while controlling for anthropometric parameters, is yet to be investigated. Knee extension concentric peak torque, jump performance, and 20 m straight-line speed were compared between age groups of under 17 (U17: $n = 24$), under 19 (U19: $n = 25$), and senior (seniors: $n = 19$) elite, national and international level, male football athletes. Analysis of covariance was performed, with height and body mass used as covariates. No significant differences were found between age groups for knee extension concentric peak torque ($p = 0.28–0.42$), while an effect was observed when the covariates of height and body mass were applied ($p < 0.001$). Senior players had greater jump and speed performance, whereas an effect was observed only for the covariate of body mass in the 15 m and 20 m ($p < 0.001$) speed testing. No differences were observed between U17 and U19 groups for jump and speed performance ($p = 0.26–0.46$). The current study suggests that younger elite football athletes (<19 years) have lower jump and speed performance than their senior counterparts, but not for strength when height and body mass are considered as covariates. Emphasis should be on power development capacities at the late youth phase when preparing athletes for the senior competition level.

Keywords: elite soccer; anaerobic alactic; age groups; performance

---

1. Introduction

An elite football (i.e., soccer) match demands a high number of short and intense activities including sprints, tackles, and jumps [1,2]. Consequently, high anaerobic abilities (e.g., maximal strength and speed) are essential factors for performance, and suggest as essential to achieve high football performance levels [1]. In elite football European clubs, a considerable number of athletes start competing at an elite level (e.g., main national division) at ages <19 years. However, it is unknown if young athletes have similar anaerobic abilities as their senior counterparts at this elite level of competition.

Previous studies have reported different strength, power, and speed characteristics between age groups in football athletes [3–6]. For instance, Kellis et al. observed a clear age effect on isokinetic concentric knee extensor strength in 158 soccer male subjects from 10 to 17 years old [6]. Also, Nikolaidis (2014) observed an age effect on lower body muscle power measured by countermovement jump [7]. This age effect on the lower body power capabilities seems to affect a wide spectrum of force–velocity muscular properties, as Nikolaidis (2012) have observed an age effect on cycling power production on both extremes of the force–velocity spectrum [8]. However, previous studies have limited their analysis to ages below the senior level [3,4,6], female populations [4], non-professional populations [5], or comparisons between competition levels [9,10]. To the best of our knowledge, no study has compared the age effects on strength, power, and speed between young and senior football athletes competing at an elite professional level. In addition, body size related parameters, such as body mass and height, have been suggested as primary contributors to explain variance in anaerobic capabilities in young football athletes [11,12]. Therefore, it is important to determine whether these anthropometric characteristics can explain potential differences in anaerobic capabilities between young and senior elite football athletes.

This study aimed to compare the differences in strength, power and speed between a group of under 17 years (U17), under 19 years (U19), and senior ($\geq$19 years) elite male football athletes, while controlling for body mass and height. We hypothesized that no differences would be seen in the anaerobic capabilities between age groups, if analysis included height and body mass as covariates.

2. Materials and Methods

2.1. Participants

Sixty-nine elite male athletes from an elite Portuguese football club were invited to participate in the study. Participants were divided in three different groups according to their age: seniors, U19, and U17. Athletes from all age groups competed at the highest national (and some international) level in football, and were familiarized with all the testing protocols and procedures before taking part in the study. During a typical training week, all age group squads had between 5 and 6 technical–tactical training sessions, and 2 and 3 resistance training sessions per week. This study followed the principles of the Declaration of Helsinki, and the local Ethics recommendations. Informed consent was obtained from each participant; and parental consent was obtained for participants under 18 years old.

2.2. Procedures

All testing was performed at the pre-season of the 2016/17 European football season. The testing sessions were performed on two consecutive days, at the same time of the day (i.e., morning). Athletes did not perform any training between testing sessions. Sprints and jump tests were performed on the first day, and the strength tests were performed on the second day. A warm-up consisting of 15-min of moderate intensity running and low intensity jumping exercises was performed at the start of each testing session.

2.3. Measures

Anthropometric measures (height and weight) were performed by the sport science and medical professionals, supervised by a member certified by the International Society for the Advancement of Kinanthropometry (ISAK). Anthropometrics measures were performed in accordance to the ISAK guidelines. Height was assessed using a stadiometer (Seca 217, Hamburg, Germany); while weight was assessed using minimal clothing and a calibrated balance ($\pm$0.1 kg, Tanita TBF 300, Tokyo, Japan).

Concentric isokinetic knee extension peak torque was assessed using an isokinetic dynamometer (Biodex System 3 research, Shirley, NY, USA) on both legs. Participants performed the testing in a seated position, while the thighs (above the knee) were stabilized by straps. The dynamometer axis was aligned with the lateral condyle of the femur. The knee range of motion limits were set between 90° and 180° (full extension). One set of six maximal knee flexion–extension (concentric/concentric) repetitions were performed for each leg at a speed of 60°/s. Torque was corrected for gravity. The peak torque output during knee extension (of each leg), measured by the Biodex software (Shirley, NY, USA, version), was used for analysis.

Vertical jump height for the countermovement jump (CMJ) followed by squat jump (SJ) and drop jump (DJ) tests was assessed using a portable optical timing system (Optojump Next; Microgate, Bolzano, Italy). Jumps were performed with the hands on the hips, and verbal encouragement was given. For the SJ, if any counter-movement action was detected by the researcher, an additional trial was performed. For the DJ, participants were required to jump from a 40-cm wooden box. Three trials were performed for each jump test (1-min rest between trials, and 5-min rest between jump tests). The best performance was used for analysis.

The time to complete 20-m in a straight-line sprint test was assessed at 5, 15, and 20 m intervals using electronic timing gates (Swift Performance SpeedLight, Queensland, Australia). The test was performed on an AstroTurf outdoor surface. Participants began each sprint from a standing position with their front foot placed 0.75 m behind the first timing gate. Participants were instructed to run as quickly as possible over the 20 m distance. Time was measured to the nearest 0.001 s. Two trials were performed, and the highest value was used for analysis.

2.4. Statistical Analysis

All data was analyzed using SPSS software (version 23.0, IBM, Chicago, IL, USA). Normal distribution was confirmed for most of independent variables using the Shapiro–Wilk test. Age, body mass, and height was compared between age groups using a one-way ANOVA followed by Bonferroni test. Analysis of strength, jumping, and speed performance between age groups were performed using one-way analysis of covariance (ANCOVA). Body mass and height were defined as covariates in the analysis. ANCOVA assumptions were confirmed using: (i) Pearson correlation coefficient between the covariates ($r < 0.8$); (ii) Levene test for determining dependent variables homogeneity; and, (iii) Shapiro–Wilk test for determining the distribution of the residuals data. When applicable, Post hoc analysis were performed using the Bonferroni test. Statistical significance was set at $p < 0.05$.

3. Results

Covariates showed a Pearson correlation coefficient lower than 0.61 for all dependent variables. Sample size, age, and anthropometric characteristics for each age group are shown in Table 1. Seniors had higher body mass than U19 ($p = 0.001$) and U17 ($p < 0.001$) groups; and were taller than the U17 group ($p = 0.01$). No differences between U19 and U17 were noted for height ($p = 0.41$) and body mass ($p = 0.92$).

Table 1. Participant characteristics. Data shown as means $\pm$ SD.

Participants Characteristics	Seniors ($n = 19$)	U19 ($n = 25$)	U17 ($n = 24$)
Age (years)	22.9 ± 4.0 #	17.4 ± 0.6 *	15.4 ± 0.8 *,#
Body Mass (kg)	78.2 ± 14.0	69.2 ± 5.0 *	67.0 ± 8.5 *
Height (cm)	181.7 ± 7.4	178.7 ± 3.8	175.9 ± 7.4 *

* Significant different compared to seniors ($p < 0.05$). # Significant different compared to U19 ($p < 0.05$).

Figure 1 presents the estimated marginal means $\pm$ standard error for all dependent variables in the different age groups. No effect was observed for age groups in knee extension concentric peak torque in both right ($p = 0.28$) and left ($p = 0.42$) limbs, except for when values were adjusted for the covariates of height (right limb: $p < 0.001$; left limb: $p < 0.001$) and body mass (right limb: $p = 0.15$; left limb: $p = 0.06$).

An effect was seen for age groups in all the jumping tests ($p < 0.001$), without a significant effect when covariates were applied (height: $p = 0.23$–0.601; body mass: $p = 0.19$–0.85). Post hoc analysis revealed that seniors had better jump performance than U19 ($p < 0.001$) and U17 ($p < 0.001$); while no differences were seen between U19 and U17 ($p = 1.00$).

Regarding sprint performance, an effect was seen for age groups in all the distances (5 m: $p = 0.004$; 15 m: $p < 0.001$; 20 m: $p < 0.001$); and an effect was observed for the body mass covariate at 15 m

($p = 0.02$) and 20 m ($p = 0.02$), with no effect for the height covariate ($p = 0.40$–0.99). Post hoc analysis revealed that seniors were faster than U19 and U17 groups for all the distances, except compared to the U19 in the 5 m distance ($p = 0.14$). No differences were observed between U19 and U17 for all sprint distances ($p = 0.26$–0.46).

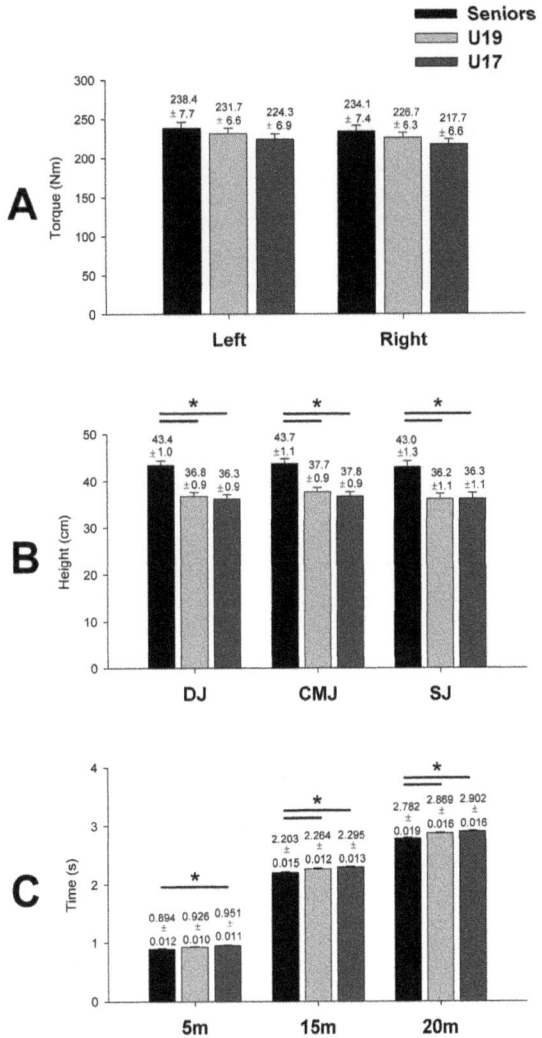

Figure 1. Estimated marginal means ± standard deviations of (**A**) knee extension peak torque of both lower limbs; (**B**) vertical jump height in three jump tests, and (**C**) sprint times at 5, 15, and 20 m for the different age groups. * $p < 0.05$. Legend: DJ; drop jump; SJ; squat jump; CMJ; countermovement jump.

4. Discussion

This study compared the anaerobic physical performance between young and senior athletes that compete at an elite level, while controlling for body mass and height. The main study findings were: (i) no differences were found between age groups for knee extension concentric peak torque, after controlling for body mass and height; (ii) jumping performance was higher for seniors compared to

U17 and U19, without influence of body mass and height; (iii) seniors were faster than younger athletes, whereas the covariate of body mass was closely related to performance at 15 and 20 m distances; and, (iv) overall, no differences were seen between U17 and U19 age groups.

The results for knee extension concentric peak torque observed in the present study were similar to those reported in previous studies examining the senior [13], U19 [5,6], and U17 [14] elite football athletes. According to our initial hypothesis, no differences were observed in knee extension concentric peak torque between age groups, when controlling for the body mass and height. This result is suggestive that the factors related to body size that affect the muscular force production may not be fully developed in athletes under 19 years old. Skeletal muscle mass, which is associated with muscle power to a greater extent than body mass [7], is a potential factor which development may not been maximized in athletes at this age; since the potential for muscle mass development is likely to still be occurring up to this age [15]. However, since we have not assessed the skeletal muscle mass, the present study does not allow us to conclude whether this factor could explain the present results, and therefore, remains speculative. Nevertheless, a potential practical implication obtained in this study is that analysis of strength performance between young and senior elite football athletes should be made by normalizing the strength to a body-size related factor, in particular to the body mass.

Moreover, previous research has suggested that some basic anthropometric characteristics, such as body mass and height, significantly contribute to explain the jumping and speed performance differences between athletes at a young age [11,12]. Thus, it would be expected that such anthropometric characteristics could explain potential performance differences between elite football athletes at a late youth phase and their senior counterparts. However, the present results do not support such rationale, since only the covariate of body mass influenced the speed at 15 m and 20 m distances. It should be noted that jumping performance has similar physiological demands than speed performance at a 5 m distance, i.e., high energy, alactic demand for a short and explosive motion involving muscular recruitment for a high rate of force production. In addition, both the jump and speed performance observed in the present study is in agreement to data of previous studies examining senior [5,10], U19 [10,16,17], and U17 [3,18] elite football athletes. Also, we observed that senior athletes presented a greater jump and speed performance than younger athletes, which suggests that these physical capacities should be considered a priority in the training of young athletes. Considering the relationship often reported between maximum strength and power [19], and since no significant effect was found for height and weight as covariates, it is possible that these anaerobic performance differences may be explained by neural factors, which may be related to maturation processes [20]. For instance, Paus et al. observed an effect of age on the increase of the axon diameter and myelination within children and adolescents [21]. These neural cell structure characteristics are known to influence action potential transmission speed [22], that contribute to the differences in short and explosive actions observed with maturation [20]. Future research is needed to examine the physiological basis of anaerobic performance deficit at this young age phase (compared to senior age groups).

5. Conclusions

In conclusion, the current study suggests that younger elite football athletes have lower jump and speed performance than their senior counterparts, but not for strength when height and body mass were considered as covariates. Based on the rationale for the development of the physical performance abilities in an athletic population [16], we would recommend that: firstly, football coaches and strength and conditioning professionals should monitor the power and strength of younger athletes in order to decide for their inclusion in senior level competition; and, secondly, priority should be given to power training for young athletes who are close to participating at a senior level of competition.

Acknowledgments: No sources of funding were used to assist in the preparation of this article.

Author Contributions: Bruno Mendes, Francisco Tavares, and Sandro Freitas conceived and designed the experiments; Bruno Mendes performed the experiments; Francisco Tavares and Sandro Freitas analyzed the data; Francisco Tavares, Matthew Driller and Sandro Freitas wrote the paper.

Conflicts of Interest: The authors declare no conflict of interest.

References

1. Stølen, T.; Chamari, K.; Castagna, C.; Wisløff, U. Physiology of soccer: An update. *Sports Med.* **2005**, *35*, 501–536. [CrossRef] [PubMed]
2. Silva, J.R.; Nassis, G.P.; Rebelo, A. Strength training in soccer with a specific focus on highly trained players. *Sports Med. Open* **2015**, *1*, 17. [CrossRef] [PubMed]
3. Le Gall, F.; Carling, C.; Williams, M.; Reilly, T. Anthropometric and Fitness Characteristics of International, Professional and Amateur Male Graduate Soccer Players from an Elite Youth Academy. *J. Sci. Med. Sport* **2010**, *13*, 90–95. [CrossRef] [PubMed]
4. Vescovi, J.D.; Rupf, R.; Brown, T.D.; Marques, M.C. Physical performance characteristics of high-level female soccer players 12–21 years of age. *Scand. J. Med. Sci. Sports* **2011**, *21*, 670–678. [CrossRef] [PubMed]
5. Dowson, M.N.; Cronin, J.B.; Presland, J.D. Anthropometric and physiological differences between gender and age groups of New Zealand National soccer players. In *Science and Football IV*; Murphy, A., Reilly, T., Spinks, W., Eds.; Routledge: Abingdon, UK, 2002; pp. 63–71. ISBN 9780415241519.
6. Kellis, S.; Gerodimos, V.; Kellis, E.; Manou, V. Bilateral isokinetic concentric and eccentric strength profiles of the knee extensors and flexors in young soccer players. *Isokinet. Exerc. Sci.* **2001**, *9*, 31–39.
7. Nikolaidis, P.T. Age-related Differences in Countermovement Vertical Jump in Soccer Players 8–31 Years Old: The Role of Fat-free Mass. *Am. J. Sports Sci. Med.* **2014**, *2*, 60–64.
8. Nikolaidis, P.T. Age-Related Differences in Force-Velocity Characteristics in Youth Soccer. *Kinesiology* **2012**, *44*, 130–138.
9. Rebelo, A.; Brito, J.; Maia, J.; Coelho-e-Silva, M.J.; Figueiredo, A.J.; Bangsbo, J.; Malina, R.M.; Seabra, A. Anthropometric characteristics, physical fitness and technical performance of under-19 soccer players by competitive level and field position. *Int. J. Sports Med.* **2013**, *34*, 312–317. [CrossRef] [PubMed]
10. Mujika, I.; Santisteban, J.; Impellizzeri, F.M.; Castagna, C. Fitness determinants of success in men's and women's football. *J. Sports Sci.* **2009**, *27*, 107–114. [CrossRef] [PubMed]
11. Malina, R.M.; Eisenmann, J.C.; Cumming, S.P.; Ribeiro, B.; Aroso, J. Maturity-associated variation in the growth and functional capacities of youth football (soccer) players 13–15 years. *Eur. J. Appl. Physiol.* **2004**, *91*, 555–562. [CrossRef] [PubMed]
12. Wong, P.-L.; Chamari, K.; Dellal, A.; Wisløff, U. Relationship between anthropometric and physiological characteristics in youth soccer players. *J. Strength Cond. Res.* **2009**, *23*, 1204–1210. [CrossRef] [PubMed]
13. Cometti, G.; Maffiuletti, N.A.; Pousson, M.; Chatard, J.-C.; Maffulli, N. Isokinetic Strength and Anaerobic Power of Elite, Subelite and Amateur French Soccer Players. *Int. J. Sports Med.* **2001**, *22*, 45–51. [CrossRef] [PubMed]
14. Iga, J.; George, K.; Lees, A.; Reilly, T. Cross-sectional investigation of indices of isokinetic leg strength in youth soccer players and untrained individuals. *Scand. J. Med. Sci. Sports* **2009**, *19*, 714–719. [CrossRef] [PubMed]
15. Faigenbaum, A.D.; Kraemer, W.J.; Blimkie, C.J.R.; Jeffreys, I.; Micheli, L.J.; Nitka, M.; Rowland, T.W. Youth resistance training: Updated position statement paper from the national strength and conditioning association. *J. Strength Cond. Res.* **2009**, *23*, S60–S79. [CrossRef] [PubMed]
16. López-Segovia, M.; Palao Andrés, J.M.; González-Badillo, J.J. Effect of 4 months of training on aerobic power, strength, and acceleration in two under-19 soccer teams. *J. Strength Cond. Res.* **2010**, *24*, 2705–2714. [CrossRef] [PubMed]
17. Comfort, P.; Stewart, A.; Bloom, L.; Clarkson, B. Relationships between strength, sprint, and jump performance in well-trained youth soccer players. *J. Strength Cond. Res.* **2014**, *28*, 173–177. [CrossRef] [PubMed]
18. Deprez, D.; Coutts, A.J.; Fransen, J.; Deconinck, F.; Lenoir, M.; Vaeyens, R.; Philippaerts, R. Relative age, biological maturation and anaerobic characteristics in elite youth soccer players. *Int. J. Sports Med.* **2013**, *34*, 897–903. [CrossRef] [PubMed]
19. Wisløff, U.; Castagna, C.; Helgerud, J.; Jones, R.; Hoff, J. Strong correlation of maximal squat strength with sprint performance and vertical jump height in elite soccer players. *Br. J. Sports Med.* **2004**, *38*, 285–288. [CrossRef] [PubMed]

20. Van Praagh, E.; France, N.M. Measuring maximal short-term power output during growth. In *Pediatric Anaerobic Performance*; Van Praagh, E., Ed.; Human Kinetics: Champaign, IL, USA, 1998; pp. 155–189.
21. Paus, T.; Zijdenbos, A.; Worsley, K.; Collins, D.L.; Blumenthal, J.; Giedd, J.N.; Rapoport, J.L.; Evans, A.C. Structural maturation of neural pathways in children and adolescents: In vivo study. *Science* **1999**, *283*, 1908–1911. [CrossRef] [PubMed]
22. Latash, M.L. *Neurophysiological Basis of Movement*; Human Kinetics: Champaign, IL, USA, 2008; ISBN 9780736063678.

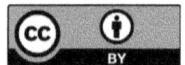

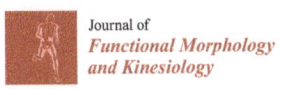

Journal of
*Functional Morphology
and Kinesiology*

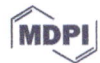

Review

The Role of Exercise in Pediatric and Adolescent Cancers: A Review of Assessments and Suggestions for Clinical Implementation

Riggs Klika [1,2], Angela Tamburini [3], Giorgio Galanti [2], Gabriele Mascherini [2] and Laura Stefani [2,*]

1   Chair American College of Sports Medicine Special Interest Group on Cancer, Sports and Exercise Medicine Center, University of Florence, Largo Brambilla 3, 50134 Florence, Italy; riggsklika@gmail.com
2   Sports and Exercise Medicine Center, Clinical and Experimental Department, School of Sports Medicine, University of Florence, Largo Brambilla 3, 50134 Florence, Italy; giorgio.galanti@unifi.it (G.G.); gabriele.mascherini@unifi.it (G.M.)
3   The Meyer Hospital, University Hospital (AOU Meyer), Viale Pieraccini 24, 50139 Firenze, Italy; angela.tamburini@meyer.it
*   Correspondence: laura.stefani@unifi.it; Tel.: +39-34-7768-9030

Received: 6 December 2017; Accepted: 10 January 2018; Published: 14 January 2018

Abstract: In the European Union, five-year survival rates for childhood cancer patients are approaching 72–80%, which is a testament to better diagnostics and improved treatment. As a result, a large proportion of childhood cancer patients go on to live productive lives well past reproductive age. While this is encouraging, childhood cancer treatment is accompanied by multiple long-term adverse effects on physical and mental wellbeing. While there are several approaches to address mental health, reproductive integrity, secondary pathologies, and recurrence, in order to optimize quality of life in childhood cancer patients, exercise and nutrition should also be considered. It is clear that physical activity plays an important role in the prevention and reduction of long-term adverse side effects associated with cancer treatment in both children and adults. However, the current exercise guidelines for cancer survivors are based on adult data and accordingly are not appropriate for children. As children and adults are markedly different, including both the pathophysiology of cancer and exercise response, treatment plans incorporating exercise for children should be age-specific and individually tailored to both reduce the development of future comorbidities and enhance physical health. The purpose of this paper is to review the predominant cancer types and effects of cancer treatment in children, describe several special considerations, and propose a framework for assessment and exercise guidelines for this population.

Keywords: cancer; children growth and maturation; physical activity; exercise; assessment

1. Introduction

The International Agency on Cancer Research estimates that, globally, 300,000 children aged 0–19 years will be diagnosed with cancer each year [1]. With current treatments, approximately 72–84% of these children will survive five or more years in the EU and USA, and to a much lesser degree (~10%) in developing countries [2–4]. While there is a disparity among survival rates in various countries, it is clear that survival rates for childhood cancer patients are improving [3]. Recent estimates from several Western countries put the proportion of long-term childhood cancer survivors (CCS) between 0.1% and 0.15% of the general population, implying that one in every 1000–1650 persons is a childhood cancer survivor [3]. In Italy about 1150 new CCS will be added to the population yearly based on an estimate that 75% of children treated on current protocols for childhood (0–19 years) cancer will become long-term survivors (>5 years) [5]. While increased survival rates are encouraging, the advancements in treatment for childhood cancer patients are unfortunately often accompanied by several late adverse events (LAE).

In children treated for cancer, LAE include impaired growth [6], cognitive dysfunction [7,8], diminished neurological function [9], cardiopulmonary compromise [10,11], musculoskeletal disturbances [10], and secondary malignancy [12,13]. As a result, adult survivors of childhood cancer may suffer from cardiomyopathy, heart valve and conduction disorders [14,15], increased cardiovascular risk factors including hypertension, dyslipidemia [16–18], and obesity [19,20], pulmonary disorders [21,22], endocrine disorders [23] including hypothalamic-pituitary-adrenal disorders [24], diabetes mellitus [25], ovarian and Leydig cell dysfunction [26], and hypothyroidism [27]. Survivors of childhood cancer are also at increased risk for neurocognitive and neurosensory impairment including ocular degeneration, hearing loss and neuropathy [28–31], metabolic disturbances (abnormal blood counts, liver and kidney dysfunction, and osteoporosis) [28–30,32,33], transfusion-associated infections [30], and increased risk of subsequent neoplasm [14]. A major concern is that chronic LAE may increase in frequency and severity over time, and interact adversely with the normal ageing process, resulting in increasing and clinically significant impairment of vital organ systems during adulthood at a younger age than normal, and an increased risk of premature major illness or death [34–37].

As with adult cancer patients, childhood cancer patients decrease their physical activity levels during and after cancer treatment, which may exacerbate LAE [10,17,36,38]. Physical activity is positively related to body weight management, cardiopulmonary fitness, musculoskeletal integrity, mental well-being, and decreased risk of premature mortality in adult cancer patients [38], while reduced physical activity is associated with decreased cardiopulmonary function, aerobic fitness, and motor-skill development/integrity and increased cachexia and cancer-related fatigue [18]. As a result of the numerous LAE related to pediatric cancer treatment, an interest in using exercise as a therapeutic measure to attenuate or reverse many cancer-related LAE in the pediatric population has surfaced. While comparatively less studied, the research suggests that there is a positive effect of physical activity on organ system function, fatigue, and physical well-being in children during and after cancer treatment [39–49]. It is clear that children who exercise can increase aerobic fitness and strength, with the latter a result of neuromuscular adaptations rather than skeletal muscle hypertrophy. The differences in the exercise training response between adults and children are most likely related to children having fairly well developed aerobic systems and relatively immature anaerobic systems [50].

What is less clear in childhood cancer patients is the physical activity level needed to increase physical function/health during and after treatment while not adding to an already elevated stress burden, which could conceivably be detrimental to the child's health. In adults, it appears that the most effective strategies for increasing physical activity levels after treatment are individualized programs that are initiated under supervision and are later adopted into life-style behaviors in an unsupervised setting [38,51]. It is not clear whether this is an ideal strategy for childhood cancer patients, but it appears that most current pediatric cancer exercise programs implement this approach [39,40].

In adult exercise oncology, the long-term strategic aim is to ensure that every cancer survivor receives optimal long-term care that increases their health and survival [38]. The goal is no different in the pediatric population [52–55], but there are much fewer data available to draw conclusive and precise exercise guidelines. Therefore, the goal of this review is to examine pediatric cancers, associated cancer treatments, and late adverse events and review emerging knowledge on pediatric exercise oncology. A summary of current exercise practices for childhood cancer patients is provided and suggestions for clinical assessment and a three-tiered rehabilitation plan are offered.

2. Types of Childhood Cancer

Childhood cancers make up less than 1% of all cancers diagnosed each year but still rank as the second-leading cause of death for children 1–14 years; they differ from adult cancer with regards to incidence and prevalence as well as etiology [2]. In children, typical cancers include acute lymphocytic leukemia (ALL) and acute myelogenous leukemia (AML), which comprise about 30% of all cancers in children [2]. ALL and AML are characterized by abnormal proliferation of leukocytes and reduction of normal blood cells. Leukemia causes bone and joint pain, fatigue, weakness, pale skin, bleeding or bruising, fever, weight loss, and other symptoms. Because acute leukemia grows quickly, chemotherapy is typically initiated soon after diagnosis.

Brain and spinal cord tumors are the second most common cancer in children, making up approximately 26% of childhood cancers. Central nervous system tumorigenesis starts in the lower parts of the brain, such as the cerebellum or brain stem, and may cause headaches, nausea, vomiting, blurred or double vision, dizziness, seizures, and trouble walking or handling objects. Spinal cord tumors are less common than brain tumors in both children and adults [2,52]. About 6% of childhood cancers are neuroblastomas, which can be found in a developing embryo or fetus. This cancer develops in infants and young children and is rarely found in children older than 10.

Wilms tumors (nephroblastoma) account for about 5% of childhood cancers and start in one, or rarely, both kidneys. They are most often found in children about 3–4 years old, and are uncommon in children older than six. They manifest as a swelling or lump in the abdomen and are characterized by fever, pain, nausea, or poor appetite.

Lymphoma (including both Hodgkin and non-Hodgkin lymphomas) starts in the lymphocytes, lymph nodes, or other lymph tissues such as the tonsils or thymus and can affect the bone marrow and other organs. Symptoms depend on where the cancer is located and can include weight loss, fever, sweats, fatigue, and swollen lymph nodes in the neck, axilla, or inguinal region. Hodgkin lymphoma accounts for about 3% of childhood cancers and is more common in early adulthood (age 15 to 40; usually people in their 20s) and late adulthood (after age 55) [2,53]. Hodgkin lymphoma is rare in children younger than five. Non-Hodgkin lymphoma makes up about 5% of childhood cancers. It is more likely to occur in younger children than Hodgkin lymphoma and is rare in children younger than three [2]. These cancers often grow quickly and require intensive treatment, but they also tend to respond better to treatment than most non-Hodgkin lymphomas in adults. Rhabdomyosarcoma is an aggressive and highly malignant form of cancer that develops from skeletal muscle cells that have failed to fully differentiate. This type of cancer can start nearly anywhere in the body, including the head and neck, groin, abdomen, pelvis, or in the appendages. It may cause pain, swelling, or both. This is the most common type of soft tissue sarcoma in children and makes up about 3% of childhood cancers [2].

Retinoblastoma is a rare cancer that develops from immature cells of the retina and accounts for about 2% of childhood cancers [2]. It usually occurs in children approximately two years old and is seldom found in children older than six. Osseous cancers (including osteosarcoma and Ewing sarcoma) account for about 3% of childhood cancers. Osteosarcoma is an aggressive malignant neoplasm of the bone that often causes bone pain that gets worse at night or with activity and produces localized swelling. Ewing sarcoma is a malignant bone tumor most often found in young teens. The most common origins of ES are the pelvis, thoracic cavity, or middle of the long leg bones [2].

3. Treatments for Childhood Cancer

Treatment for childhood cancer is based on the type and stage of the cancer. Types of treatment used for childhood cancer include: surgery, chemotherapy, radiation, hormone therapy, stem cell transplantation, and newer treatments such as targeted drug therapy and immunotherapy. Often, multiple treatments are indicated. Chemotherapy for CCS includes alkylating agents, antimetabolites, anthracyclines, plant alkaloids, antitumor antibiotics, taxanes, and monoclonal antibodies. Childhood cancers usually respond well to high-dose chemotherapy because of rapid cell turnover in children and are effective but often lead to more short- and long-term side effects [2]. In general, the more frequently recognized risk factors for long-term events in children include patient age at treatment, cumulative treatment dose, and the treatment schedule of radio- or chemotherapy [13,54].

4. Late Adverse Events (LAE) in Childhood Cancer Patients

The high survival rate in children and adolescents with malignancy is accompanied by a substantial risk of late adverse events (LAE) as a result of long-term radio- and chemotherapy. Chemotherapy for pediatric cancer suppresses the immune system and may interfere with normal growth, increasing susceptibility to infection and stunting or delaying musculoskeletal development during treatment [49]. Treatments may interfere with physiological growth and development in children and adolescents and have an important impact on health status later in life, while some late toxicities (e.g., pulmonary fibrosis, obesity, hypertension, cardiovascular disease) may cause premature death [11,14,16,17,20,21,25,28,31]. It has been estimated that 62% of adult survivors of childhood malignancy have ≥1, and 38% ≥2, treatment-induced chronic health conditions, and 28% a severe or life-threatening problem such as cardiomyopathy [30]. Survivors of central nervous system tumors or hematopoietic stem cell transplantation are at particularly high risk [8,30].

5. Complications after Childhood/Adolescent Cancer Treatment

CCS are potentially vulnerable to a variety of long-term therapy-related complications, and therefore lifestyle management is important in reducing LAE commonly present during adulthood. Physical and psychosocial adverse treatment effects can increase premature morbidity and mortality when compared to the general population, and therefore developing strategies for long-term follow-up of survivors of childhood cancer is essential [29,48].

Among the most serious health complications in CCS following treatment are pulmonary and heart disorders [3,30]. Chronic pulmonary disease is the number one LAE following childhood cancer treatment, with 65.2% of those followed up having abnormal pulmonary function [30]. Bleomycin toxicity resulting in pulmonary fibrosis, radiation to the lungs, thoracotomy, and busulfan treatment increase the risk of abnormal pulmonary function in CCS. Both restrictive and obstructive lung disease may occur, while bronchiectasis may result from previous lower respiratory tract infections.

Cardiac abnormalities have been reported in 56% of survivors of childhood cancer treatment, who are 5–15 times more likely to experience heart disease than their siblings [17,30,44]. The major risk factors for the development of cardiac dysfunction are treatment with anthracyclines and/or radiotherapy to the heart. Vinca alkaloids and alkylating agents have also been implicated in cardiovascular complications, along with young age at treatment, female gender, and length of follow-up. Chemotherapy and radiotherapy increase cardiovascular disease in the form of coronary artery damage, myocardial failure, pericardial disease, valvular abnormalities, conduction disorders, and increased cardiovascular risk factors. Valvular regurgitation is common (56%) in adult survivors of childhood cancer who have been previously exposed to radiotherapy, while systolic dysfunction is prevalent after exposure to anthracyclines or both treatments (6%) [17]. Fifty percent of CCS reported being obese, 61% have dyslipidemia, and 23% are hypertensive—all increasing the risk of future cardiovascular disease [30].

In CCS, as well as adults who are survivors of childhood cancer, the risk of clinical metabolic syndrome is high [26]. Metabolic syndrome (MS) is characterized by a clustering of hypertension, dyslipidemia, type 2 diabetes or preclinical conditions, and obesity. MS is associated with a proinflammatory and pro-thrombotic state that may lead to atherogenic dyslipidemia. There is evidence that survivors exposed to cranial radiotherapy, prolonged steroid treatment, total body or abdominal irradiation, and those with hypogonadism or limitations in physical performance are at increased risk of glucose intolerance and MS.

Cancer treatment is also related to several acute or chronic renal complications. Nephrotoxicity may be due to glomerular or tubular damage, or both. Renal failure or the requirement for dialysis is an uncommon but serious late complication, occurring in <1%, but with a relative risk ratio estimated at about 8 [35]. The main risk factors for nephrotoxicity are the specific chemotherapy drugs received. For example, ifosfamide nephrotoxicity is more common in patients treated with a cumulative dose

>80 g·m^{-2}. Platinum nephrotoxicity is more common in children treated with a higher cisplatin dose rate (>40 mg·m^{-2}·day^{-1}) or higher cumulative carboplatin doses and those treated at an older age.

Endocrine complications are similar in overall prevalence to cardiac abnormalities in CCS, occurring in 20–50% of survivors followed into adulthood [30]. Complications include hypothalamo-pituitary, thyroid, and gonadal dysfunction, bone disease, and metabolic disorders, which are associated with the tumor type and location and treatment. In addition to the effects of surgery or direct endocrine gland involvement by the malignancy, both radio- and chemotherapy may increase the risk of endocrine complications involving several glands. These are the most frequently reported complications of childhood cancer survivors, affecting between 20% and 50% of individuals who survive into adulthood. Most endocrine complications are the result of prior cancer treatments, especially radiotherapy. Survivors treated with radiotherapy to the head, neck, or pelvis, and those treated with total body irradiation or with alkylating agents, are at increased risk. Growth hormone deficiency is the most common anterior pituitary deficiency observed after standard cranial radiotherapy. It may manifest after a standard cranial radiotherapy dose $\geq$18 Gy; >24 Gy the deficiency usually manifests within five years, while for doses in the range of 18–24 Gy the deficiency may become manifest after 10–15 years [49]. Other endocrine disorders in CCS include precocious puberty in young females treated for ALL, which is related to radiation of the hypothalmo-pituitary axis in the range 18–24 Gy.

Ovarian germ cell failure and loss of ovarian endocrine function occur concomitantly in females [10,13,15,30]. They may be due to pelvic, abdominal, or spinal radiation, total body irradiation, or alkylating agent chemotherapy. Age at treatment is important in predicting ovarian failure, since females treated at a younger age are less likely to develop ovarian failure, probably because of a higher number of primordial follicles at the time of treatment. Uterine morphology should be evaluated in females treated with pelvic or abdominal radiation, to assess the likelihood of embryonal implantation or completion of fetal development. The testis is sensitive both to chemotherapy and radiation [23]. Among chemotherapeutic agents, cumulative doses of alkylating agents and timing of treatment influence the risk of oligo/azoospermia. Damage to the germinal epithelium is estimated to occur after a testicular dose <1.2 Gy either as direct testicular radiotherapy or during abdominal or spinal radiation or an inverted Y field for Hodgkin disease (HD) treatment. Leydig cells are much more radioresistant and only doses >20 Gy (pre-pubertal patients) or >30 Gy (post-pubertal individuals) may result in complete primary hypogonadism. In contrast to females, age at treatment has minimal impact on testicular function.

The thyroid gland is sensitive to radiotherapy given either externally to the neck or targeted via thyroid metabolism. The functional changes after external beam radiation usually occur by six months but may become evident up to 20 years later, and comprise clinical or subclinical hypothyroidism, with a combined incidence of 20–30% [6,7,16]. The morphological changes consist of benign lesions, primarily adenomas, and malignant lesions, with an average 6-fold increased risk compared to the normal population. The effect of radiotherapy on the thyroid gland is dose- and age-dependent, with younger children at a higher risk. A linear relationship with radiotherapy doses and late thyroid complications has been observed, but after doses >30 Gy the cancer risk decreases, probably because of a cell-killing effect.

Long-term neurological toxicity is a common late adverse event reported in some large CCS cohorts, occurring in 27% of survivors, with a relative risk ratio of 3.3 compared to a sibling control group. CCS with central nervous system tumors are at the highest risk, followed by survivors of Hodgkin disease or acute leukemia [18]. There are several manifestations of central nervous system toxicity, including leukoencephalopathy, vasculopathy, radiation necrosis, myelopathy, and secondary tumors, with a wide variety of clinical sequelae threatening life or greatly impairing the survivor's quality of life. Neurocognitive impairment is common in CCS being reported as high as 48% [30]. Other impairments include ocular (28%), vestibular/hearing loss (62%), and neuropathy (22%) [54]. The major cause of deafness in survivors of childhood malignancy is platinum chemotherapy. Both higher cumulative cisplatin dose and younger age at treatment predict a higher risk of deafness, with a total dose

> 400 mg·m^{-2} and age <5 years associated with development of bilateral sensorineural hearing loss in 40% of children. The consequences of deafness in children include delayed speech development and impaired educational/social functioning, especially in younger children.

Specific treatment-related complications occur in very young cancer patients. Craniofacial and dental complications are more prevalent in patients treated at a young age. The younger the child and the higher the radiation dose, the more pronounced the growth impairment. Radiotherapy to the face or brain may lead to hypoplasia of the irradiated area. As normal growth occurs, the deformity becomes progressively more pronounced. However, the most evident effect on linear growth is seen when radiotherapy is given before skeletal maturation has occurred [7]. Bone irradiation >20 Gy, especially near long-bone growth plates, leads to reduced bone growth and potentially asymmetric limb growth. If the spine is involved in the radiation field, vertebral bodies will display impaired growth, leading to a reduced adult height, with disproportion between standing and sitting height [32]. Scoliosis may result from soft tissue fibrosis secondary to radiotherapy to paravertebral tissues/organs. Avascular necrosis of bone may occur either during or after therapy, particularly with radiation and/or prolonged steroid treatment, and usually affects joints in long bones, causing pain and functional impairment.

Survivors of hematopoietic stem cell transplant (HSCT) are at particularly high risk of late adverse complications, with >90% suffering from at least one and >70% from at least three chronic conditions [8]. Patients treated with total body irradiation are at the highest risk of late toxicity, and high-dose chemotherapy is an additional potent risk factor. Additive and potentially synergistic damage results from numerous other factors, including previous treatment given before transplant, the development of other serious complications after HSCT, potentially toxic supportive care drugs, and especially chronic graft vs. host–disease, which may affect any organ, tissue, or body system. Chronic graft versus host–disease occurs in up to 30% of HSCT patients, with multiple potential sequelae including organ and tissue damage, as well as functional impairment and the potential adverse effects of immunosuppressive drugs.

Surgical complications and late physical effects must be considered in CCS. Orthopedic treatment for cancer may result in partial or total bone damage and prosthetic implantation [15]. As a result of surgery, posture, gait, and physical activity levels are affected [32]. The management of the correct/neutral posture and proper motor skill development need to be emphasized and eventually modified to follow the disease progression. Although the quality of life of these surgical patients in domains other than physical functioning is as high as that seen in controls, there is a life-long need for many patients to have continued contact with health services, e.g., for prosthetic reasons or post-surgical complications.

Last, the psychosocial consequences of childhood cancer and LAE should be considered. It is clear that psychological or social consequences interfere with quality of life (QoL), which comprises elements of physical, functional, social, and psychological health [21,22,47,55–58]. QoL may be affected by the level of integration into society, as measured by the survivors' probability (compared to age and sex-matched general population peers) of securing employment or health insurance, or of marrying [57]. It is important that the public ensures that cancer survivors have equal access to education, jobs, insurance, and medical care. The Children's Oncology Group (COG) www.survivorshipguidelines.org has developed long-term follow-up guidelines for survivors of childhood cancers [59]; however, a specific path for the transition from hospital-based care to home-based rehabilitation has not been clearly defined.

6. Guidelines for Assessment

The choice of assessment protocols for CCS depends on the specific questions that one may ask and, as a rule, one should test those physiological functions that are most likely to yield relevant clinical and functional information. A summary of potential test battery items is presented in Table 1. At a minimum, practitioners should be regularly measuring body dimensions including stature, weight, head circumference, and an index of body composition (e.g., BMI, skinfolds at four sites (triceps, biceps, subscapular and iliac crest, and circumferences (arm relaxed and flexed, calf) for muscle mass development)) following international standards measurement sites and procedures [60,61]. Comparisons can be made by sex, and to population-specific normative data. Tracking changes in stature, weight, weight-to-stature ratio, and body mass index will provide insight into nutritional status and normal body growth [62]. Body composition analysis using bioelectrical impedance or DXA scanning may provide more detailed information on total body water distribution and fat versus fat-free mass components; however, due to the large variability in body composition during growth, the clinical use of these tools is questionable. Additionally, errors in interpreting DXA results may generate considerable parental concern and can result in costly and unnecessary use of pharmacologic agents and restrictions on physical activity [63].

Table 1. Potential assessment items for pediatric cancer patients.

Domain Being Measured	Item
Body size and nutritional status	Height (cm) Weight (kg) BMI Head Circumference Skinfolds (mm)
Motor Skill	Posture Gait Balance Motor skill proficiency
Flexibility	Sit and Reach Ankle dorsiflexion
Performance Level	Hand grip dynamometry (kg) TUG-3 m (s) 30 s Chair stand (# of successful stands)
Cardiovascular Fitness	PWC_{150} Echocardiography CPET (VO_2 peak) ($mL \cdot kg^{-1} \cdot min^{-1}$)
Pulmonary Function	Spirometry (FEV, FEV_1)
Quality of Life	PCQL Inventory

References for each test item can be found in the text. TUG: timed get up and go; PWC: power work capacity; FEV: forced expiratory volume, FEV1: forced expiratory volume in 1 sec, PCQL: pediatric cancer quality of life.

7. Echocardiographic Assessment

Echocardiography represents the best non-invasive method for obtaining sufficient information in CCS as part of a complete clinical evaluation to clear the patient for physical activity. Echocardiographic stress testing is considered the standard of care in contemporary assessment regarding left ventricular performance, pulmonary pressure measurement, and valve behavior, and should be considered for all CCS [30,31,64]. In addition to the standard echocardiographic measures (i.e., systolic and diastolic data of the left and right ventricles), velocity parameters (tissue velocity imaging or TDI) and deformation measures (strain) are now routinely used in the assessment and management of cancer patients participating in regular physical activity and more strenuous sports [64–68]. Echocardiography, as an advanced tool in cardio-oncology, can be used to detect early-stage myocardial damage and its applications are now being used in the pediatric population [68].

7.1. Cardiopulmonary Exercise Testing (CPET)

In healthy children, or those with a cardiopulmonary disease, cardiopulmonary exercise testing is considered the gold standard for assessing aerobic fitness and when equipment accommodations should be made for the child (e.g., smaller cycle ergometer, child-specific graded exercise protocols) [50]. CPET is both reliable and valid in the pediatric population [69]. CPET can provide information about aerobic fitness, hemodynamic response to exercise, metabolic response, and ventilatory thresholds. Data obtained from symptom-limited CPET are sufficient to establish exercise intensity guidelines for CCS. Variables measured during CPET include electrocardiogram, power or workload (speed and grade), heart rate, oxygen saturation, blood pressure, and a rating of perceived exertion (RPE). A Borg scale of 6–20 or modified Borg scale of 1–10 can be used to evaluate RPE [70]. Post-CPET, monitoring should be continued for 5–10 min and terminated when the heart rate has returned to 110% (or lower) of the pre-exercise testing heart rate.

7.2. Power Work Capacity (PWC$_{150}$)

Power work capacity is a submaximal cycle ergometer test whereby the child is asked to pedal a cycle ergometer at a specific power that will elicit a heart rate of 150 beats·min^{-1}. Power is recorded as the outcome measure. Changes in PWC$_{150}$ reflect cardiovascular fitness and can be administered on a regular basis without the specialized metabolic analyzers needed for CPET [69].

7.3. Pulmonary Function Testing (PFT)

PFT should include spirometry that measures forced vital capacity (FVC) and forced expiratory volume in 1 s (FEV$_1$) in order to screen for restrictive or obstructive airway disease caused by radiation and pulmonary fibrosis. Preliminary screening should be followed by referral to pediatric pulmonary specialists if abnormal values are detected and prior to the CCS participating in structured physical activity.

7.4. Motor and Skill Assessment

As a component of physical function, an age-appropriate motor skill assessment should be made. In children 0–2 years of age, the Bayley Infant Scoring system for neurocognitive development has been routinely used and is both reliable and valid [71]. If the child has developed basic movement skills (walk, run, throw, skip, hop, leap) then an assessment of fundamental movement skills may be appropriate [72,73]. Nauman et al. have reported the performance efficiency on the sprint run, vertical jump, side gallop, leap, catch, kick, and overarm throw efficacy in childhood cancer patients, which discriminated between oncology patients and health controls [72].

Posture and gait analysis will provide information on orthopedic dysfunction, equilibrium, skeletal musculoskeletal integrity, and neuromotor processing and activation. Visual inspection and scoring of posture by a trained specialist is warranted and observational gait analysis or videography may be used in the determination of abnormal/normal gait mechanics [74]. Videography provides a permanent record of the child's performance that can subsequently digitally analyzed for quantitative evaluation of the patient. There are no standards for posture and gait analysis in pediatric cancer patients.

Flexibility can be assessed using a modified sit and reach test, but there is large experimental error with this measure. Additionally, ankle dorsiflexion with goniometers has been measured in children to assess lower limb extremity extensibility for proper foot mechanics [39].

Strength: As a proxy for total body strength, hand grip dynamometry has been used extensively. It requires minimal equipment and provides an estimation of overall strength. Other performance measures used in the pediatric cancer population include the timed get up and go test (TUG) and the 30 s chair test [40]. Both provide information on strength and neuromuscular coordination.

7.5. Quality of Life (QoL)

Quality of life in both childhood and adult cancer patients has been well researched and there are a number of validated age-specific scales designed to assess the emotional, physical, and social aspects of one's life [21,45,53,56–58]. As part of a comprehensive rehabilitation plan for CCS, the authors support the importance of QoL assessment as part of the rehabilitation plan. The Pediatric Cancer Quality of Life Inventory is specific to this population and is a reliable tool [58].

7.6. Nutrition

Nutrition plays a critical role in normal growth and maturation and the client's diet should be ascertained during cancer treatment and age-appropriate nutritional guidelines for weight gain or to control obesity should be conveyed to the CCS caregiver [43–45]. Clinical dietitians are encouraged to be part of the pediatric cancer care team. Specifics of nutritional concerns for CCS are beyond the scope of this paper and are purposefully omitted.

8. Guidelines for Exercise Prescription in Pediatric Cancer Patients

Braam et al. provide the most current review of childhood and young adult cancer exercise training interventions during and after cancer [39]. In general, children need a minimal level of physical fitness for normal growth and development [50]. As cancer treatment often interrupts structured and unstructured physical activity during treatment, and physical activity and motor proficiency both during and after treatment have been shown to increase physical and mental wellbeing outcomes in childhood cancer patients, is seems reasonable to suggest that childhood cancer patients should engage in some physical activity during treatment and strive to reduce sedentary behavior. The extent of the physical activity is dependent on age, type of cancer and stage, and type of treatment and limitations caused by the disease itself or treatment complications [40]. For children who are extremely frail (osteopenic, immunosuppressed, low cardiorespiratory fitness), adjustments to the recommendations will need to be considered (less time, lower intensity and frequency, and smaller workloads).

Accordingly, the frequency, intensity, time, and type (FITT) of exercise used for healthy children may not apply to this population. Of the few studies published on exercise programs for childhood cancer patients, a combination of home-based (2× per week) and clinically based (hospital) programs (1× per week) for approximately 60 min per session appears to work well [27,37–40,43,47]. For children who may not be able to attend a supervised exercise training session, home-based, parent-supervised exercise is considered appropriate [39,40]. It is important to note that parents of childhood cancer patients should be instructed on appropriate exercises and contraindications for their child and encouraged to participate with the child when exercising at home.

Exercise programs for childhood cancer patients in randomized control trials have both aerobic and resistance/strength training components [40]. Aerobic or endurance training appears to be tolerable with few adverse outcomes at a moderate intensity of 50–70% age-predicted maximal heart rate for approximately 20 min/session [40]. Resistance training in childhood cancer patients has consisted of traditional gym training equipment and a combination of 11–12 movements targeting major muscle groups (bench press, leg extension leg curl, shoulder press, leg press, abdominal crunch, arm curl, back extension, seated row, latissimus pulldown) [39,40]. Accommodations for children must be made when using exercise equipment designed for adults including proper body alignment within the machine, smaller free weights (less than 1 kg), and proper supervision to ensure child safety.

9. Recommendations

In CCS, exercise training may be separated into three distinct phases with the understanding that the phases may overlap given the complexity of treatment, complications, and severity of the disease. The three-phase pediatric rehabilitation is presented schematically in Figure 1. Exercise guidelines for healthy children include the goal of 60 min of daily moderate to vigorous activity [75]; however, the duration and frequency in pediatric cancer patients will vary considerably. In phase I or ongoing treatment, it is suggested that exercise should be conservative and supervised. Medical oncology clearance for participation in structured activity is critical. In the early phase of exercise prescription, moving from sedentary behavior to any movement is the primary goal. This exercise may include walking under supervision, physical-therapy-assisted strength training or rehabilitation exercises following surgery. Aerobic exercise duration for CCS may start as low as 5–10 min daily based on health condition and progress with modest increases in session duration (e.g., 5 min). Duration of exercise should be increased prior to increasing intensity of exercise and once a minimum of 30 min of continuous activity at low intensity is feasible, exercise intensity can be increased. Peak aerobic exercise intensity should be determined based on symptom-limited echocardiographic stress data. Most studies on exercise intensity for CCS are based on percentages of maximal heart rate (50–70+% HR_{max}) [39,40]. In the absence of a peak exercise evaluation, exercise should start at 40–60% of heart rate reserve (HRR), using age-predicted maximal heart rates. As there is high variability in age-predicted maximal heart rates, adjustment to the exercise intensity should be made during the initial week of training. In the absence of any heart rate data, the use of RPE is relatively simple to use to gauge the intensity of exercise. Children should be encouraged to work at an intensity level between 1 and 5 on a 10-point RPE scale and not to exceed a level 6 during this phase. Heart rates corresponding to the appropriate RPE level can then be used in subsequent exercise sessions. Our approach to exercise intensity is somewhat conservative relative to other exercise trials in pediatric cancer patients but should be considered in the context of our health care model. Prior to each exercise session, the child should be adequately hydrated and properly nourished, and should avoid exercising in a hypoglycemic state. Additional considerations for testing and exercise training are presented in Table 2.

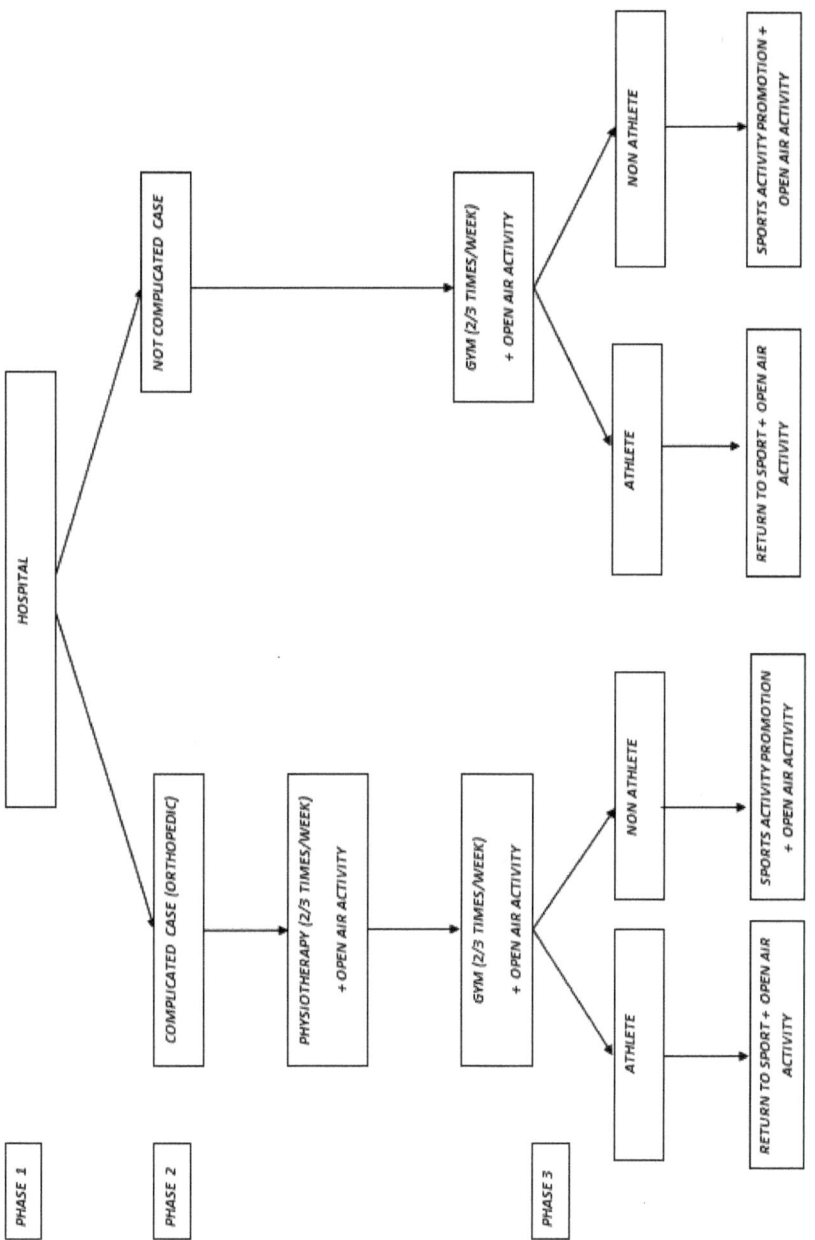

Figure 1. Flow-chart of the three-phase pediatric cancer rehabilitation.

Table 2. Contraindications and precautions to exercise testing and training for patients with cancer.

Considerations	Contraindications to Exercise Testing and Training	Precautions Requiring Modification and/or Physician Approval
Factors Related to Cancer Treatment	No exercise on days of intravenous chemotherapy (recommendation changing) No exercise before blood draw Severe tissue reaction to radiation therapy	Caution if on treatments that affect the lung and/or heart: recommend medically supervised exercise testing and training Mouth sores/ulcerations: avoid mouthpiece for maximal testing: use face mask Lymphedema: wear appropriate compression garments
Hematologic	Platelet Count <50,000 Hemoglobin level <10.0 g/dL Absolute Neutrophil Count <0.5 × 10^9/L	Platelets >50,000–150,000: avoid tests or exercise (contact sports) that increase risk of bleeding White blood cells >3000–4000: ensure proper sterilization of equipment Hemoglobin >10 g/dL—11.5–13.5 g/dL: caution with maximal tests Avoid activities that may increase the risk of bacterial infection (swimming)
Musculoskeletal	Extreme fatigue/muscle weakness Bone, back or neck pain Severe cachexia (loss of >35% premorbid weight) Karnofsky performance status score <60%; Poor functional status: avoid exercise testing	Any pain or cramping: investigate Osteopenia: avoid high-impact exercise if risk of fracture Loss of muscle mass limits exercise to mild intensity Cachexia: multidisciplinary approach to exercise
Systemic	Acute infections Febrile illness: fever >100 F General Malaise	May indicate systemic infection and should be investigated. Avoid high intensity exercise Avoid exercise until asymptomatic for >48 h
Gastrointestinal	Severe Nausea Dehydration Vomiting or diarrhea within 24–36 h Poor nutrition: inadequate fluid and/or intake	Compromised fluid and/or food intake: recommend multidisciplinary approach/consultation with nutritionist Ensure adequate nutrition with electrolyte drinks and water (avoid hyponatremia)
Cardiovascular	Chest pain Resting HR >100 bpm or <50 bpm Resting SBP >145 mm Hg and/or DBP >95 mm Hg Resting SBP <85 mm Hg Irregular HR Swelling of ankles	Exercise is contraindicated (refer to physician) Caution: recommend medically supervised exercise testing and training Exercise is contraindicated (refer to physician) Lymphedema: wear appropriate compression garments
Pulmonary	Dyspnea Cough, wheezing Chest pain increased by deep breath	Mild to moderate dyspnea: avoid maximal tests Avoid activities that require significant oxygen transport (high intensity X)
Neurologic	Ataxia/Dizziness/peripheral Sensory Neuropathy Significant decline in cognitive performance Disorientation Blurred vision	Avoid activities that require significant balance and coordination (treadmill) Ensure patient is able to understand and follow instructions Use well supported positions for exercise

Adapted from McNeely et al. [76]. HR: heart rate; SBP: systolic blood pressure; DBP: diastolic blood pressure.

Resistance training programs for CCS include body weight calisthenics, games of tag or wolf, obstacle course runs, and simple gymnastics. Emphasis should be placed on total body awareness and proprioceptive feedback. The primary goal in the initial phase of exercise prescription for CCS is to make the activity fun and promote motor skill development as motor skill proficiency is related to increased lifetime physical activity [77]. The programs need not be performance-based and careful instruction on movement patterns should be encouraged [72]. Adherence to specific sets and repetitions should be encouraged, while fatigue and improper postural alignment or biomechanics should serve as an indicator to terminate the specific exercise. Once proper movement patterns can be maintained for a specific exercise through an entire set of repetitions, the workload can then be increased either by adding more resistance or adding more repetitions per set.

In phase II, the CCS is moving from hospital-based exercise (professionally supervised) to a mixed home-based and parent-supervised program with the goal of ensuring patient stability. In phase II, aerobic conditioning duration should be extended from 30 to 45 min (multiple sessions per day is allowable) and each session should include a 5-min warm-up session and 5-min cooldown period at low intensity. The remainder of the session is designed to elicit a heart rate of 50–85% of peak exercise intensity determined at patient discharge. This corresponds to levels 1–7 on a 10-point RPE scale but no higher. In phase II, children should be encouraged to continue strength training (rehabilitation from orthopedic surgery or to correct muscle imbalances), add flexibility exercises where needed, and continue with sports specific motor skill development. Trial and error in motor skill development in the form of play is recommended and activities should be designed to be age-appropriate, entertaining, and fun. Gymnastics, swimming, and team sports (with precautions taken for contact sports) should be encouraged if the child is interested.

In phase III (at approximately 6–12 months post-discharge), CCS should be encouraged to participate in regular exercise for health maintenance or be cleared for regular sports participation. Clearance to move into competitive sports should be made by the oncology team and assessments made by Sports Medicine physicians. For those moving into competitive sports, assessment of mobility, joint stability, and movement patterns, followed by increased strength training, is recommended. Time dedicated to specific sports practice will then need to be individually determined.

In all three rehabilitation phases (hospital-based training, transition to home-based training, and competitive sports training), documentation of training should encouraged. A daily log of exercise should be maintained and relayed on a regular basis to the sports medicine team for review and ongoing adjustments to the exercise plan. Assessments should be made at the time of hospital discharge and after six and 12 months. A summary of each phase of the pediatric exercise rehabilitation plan is presented in Table 3.

Table 3. Summary of phase I–III pediatric cancer rehabilitation.

Phase	Where	Assessment	Exercise Plan	Comments
I	Hospital Based	Anthropometry: height, weight, BMI, head circumference, skinfolds and muscle circumferences. Consult with dietitian and oncology team if patient appears malnourished.	Hospital based under supervision.	Training plan: Emphasis on fundamental movements patterns (motor skill) and fun
		Orthopedic evaluation: Abnormal: refer to pediatric orthopedic team.		Modality: play (if possible), walking, cycle ergometer, stretching.
		Look for any obvious swellings or surgical scars.		Frequency 2–5x per week
		Assess for deformity: scoliosis, kyphosis, loss of lumbar lordosis or hyperlordosis of the lumbar spine. Look for shoulder asymmetry and pelvic tilt. Postural scoliosis resolves on bending, structural scoliosis does not resolve.		Intensity: Low–to moderate HR
		Observe the patient walking to assess for any abnormalities of gait.		Duration: 5–60 min per session depending on status
		Cardiopulmonary Exercise Testing (CPET)—Cycle ergometry, ECG, O_2 saturation, HR, RPE.		Play: balance, agility, hopping, skipping, throwing
		Power work capacity: Work capacity at Heart rate of 150 bpm		Routine: Warm up exercises with body weight, play or aerobic exercise, strength exercises, cool down.
		Pulmonary function testing: Spirometry		Monitor HR, O_2 saturation if needed, dyspnea, RPE, fatigue level
		Motor skill: Gait, Time up and go		
		Flexibility: sit and reach		
		Strength: Hand grip dynamometry, 30 s chair stand		
		Quality of Life: PedQoL		
II	Transition to Home based	Assessment: Nurse, physical therapist, psychologist, cancer specialist in addition to medical team	Home-based under parental supervision.	Training plan: Emphasis on aerobic fitness, fundamental movements patterns (motor skill) and fun
		Anthropometry: height, weight, BMI, head circumference, skinfolds and muscle circumferences. Consult with dietitian and oncology team if patient appears malnourished.		Goal: return to normal activities and sport activities
		Power work capacity: Work capacity at Heart rate of 150 bpm		Modality: play (if possible), walking, cycle ergometer, stretching.
		Pulmonary function testing: Spirometry		Frequency: 3–5x per week
		Motor skill: Gait, TUG		Intensity: Low–to moderate HR
		Flexibility: sit and reach	Education materials for parents and siblings.	Duration: 20–60 min per session depending on status
		Strength: Hand grip dynamometry, 30 s chair stand		Play: balance, agility, hopping, skipping, throwing
				Routine: Warm up exercises with body weight, play or aerobic exercise, strength exercises, cool down.
				Monitor HR and complete home exercise log.
III	Home based and Independent	Assessment at 6 months and 12 months, 5, 10, 15 years (in addition to medical team)	Home-based no supervision	Emphasis on strength, proficiency, postural control, cardiovascular conditioning and fun
		Anthropometry: height, weight, BMI, head circumference, skinfolds and muscle circumferences.		Goal: return to normal activities and sport activities
		Power work capacity: Work capacity at Heart rate of 150 bpm		Modality: play (if possible), walking, cycle ergometer, stretching, sports activities.
		Pulmonary function testing: Spirometry		Frequency: 3–5x per week
		Motor skill: Gait, TUG		Intensity: Low, moderate and vigorous HR
		Flexibility: sit and reach		Duration: 30–60 min per session depending on status
		Strength: Hand grip dynamometry, 30-s chair stand		Play: team sports (football), swimming.
				Routine: Warm up exercises with body weight, play or aerobic exercise, strength exercises, cool down.
				Monitor HR and complete home exercise log.

10. Conclusions

The purpose of this paper was to present a review of childhood cancer types, associated cancer treatments, and late adverse events. The second aim was to suggest pediatric-specific assessments for childhood cancer patients in order to aid in the development of appropriate therapeutic exercise programs. The third aim was to outline a three-phased rehabilitation plan for childhood cancer patients. Contraindications and precautions for exercise testing and participation were also presented.

The population of childhood cancer survivors is likely to increase in the future and an important component of their treatment should be to optimize quality of life and reduce late adverse events by using exercise as a medicine. Research in pediatric oncology has clearly shown the positive impact of exercise interventions both during and after cancer treatment. In order to provide safe and efficacious exercise programs for childhood cancer patients, a multifactorial approach is necessary, which should include input from oncology and pediatric specialists from multiple disciplines: orthopedics, cardiology, endocrinology, pulmonology, sports medicine, psychology, nutrition, and exercise oncology specialists.

In order to provide pediatric oncology patients with safe programs, we propose a three-phase rehabilitation plan whereby phase I should be initiated in the hospital setting with physical therapists and cancer exercise specialists working in collaboration with the entire pediatric medical oncology team. In phase I rehabilitation for childhood cancer patients, the goal of increasing physical activity, avoiding sedentary behavior with an emphasis on motor skill acquisition, is paramount. Following patient discharge, in phase II rehabilitation (home-based exercise) a shift to aerobic, strength, flexibility, and motor skill refinement is the main goal and will require parental education and exercise supervision. In phase III (independent, unsupervised, or team sports) will require the involvement of parents, coaches, and regional specialists to successfully monitor the child's athletic development.

Conflicts of Interest: The authors declare no conflict of interest.

References

1. Steliarova-Foucher, E.; Colombet, M.; Ries, L.A.G.; Moreno, F.; Dolya, A.; Bray, F.; Hesseling, P.; Shin, H.Y.; Stiller, C.A. International incidence of childhood cancer, 2001–10: A population-based registry study. *Lancet Oncol.* **2017**, *18*, 719–731. [CrossRef]
2. American Cancer Society. *Cancer Facts & Figures 2016*; American Cancer Society: Atlanta, GA, USA, 2016.
3. Gatta, G.; Botta, L.; Rossi, S.; Aareleid, T.; Bielska-Lasota, M.; Clavel, J.; Dimitrov, N.; Jakab, Z.; Kaatsch, P.; Lacour, B.; et al. The EUROCARE Working Group Childhood cancer survival in Europe 1999–2007: Results of EUROCARE-5—A population based study. *Lancet Oncol.* **2014**, *15*, 35–47. [CrossRef]
4. Howlader, N.; Noone, A.M.; Krapcho, M.; Miller, D.; Bishop, K.; Kosary, C.L.; Yu, M.; Ruhl, J.; Tatalovich, Z.; Mariotto, A.; et al. (Eds.) *SEER Cancer Statistics Review, 1975–2014*; National Cancer Institute: Bethesda, MD, USA. Available online: https://seer.cancer.gov/csr/1975_2014/ (accessed on 4 April 2017).
5. Mosso, M.L.; Colombo, R.; Giordano, L.; Pastore, G.; Terracini, B.; Magnani, C. Childhood cancer registry of the province of Torino, Italy: Survival, incidence and mortality over 20 years. *Cancer* **1992**, *69*, 1300–1306. [CrossRef] [PubMed]
6. Armstrong, G.T.; Chow, E.J.; Sklar, C.A. Alterations in pubertal timing following therapy for childhood malignancies. In *Endocrinopathy after Childhood Cancer Treatment*; Wallace, W.H.B., Kelnar, C.J.H., Eds.; Karger Publishers: Basel, Switzerland, 2009; Volume 15, pp. 25–39.
7. Armstrong, G.T.; Stovall, M.; Robison, L.L. Long-term effects of radiation exposure among adult survivors of childhood cancer: Results from the Childhood Cancer Survivor Study. *Radiat. Res.* **2010**, *174*, 840–850. [CrossRef] [PubMed]
8. Bhatia, S.; Davies, S.M.; Baker, S.K.; Pulsipher, M.A.; Hansen, J.A. NCI, NHLBI first international consensus conference on late effects after pediatric hematopoietic cell transplantation: Etiology and pathogenesis of late effects after HCT performed in childhood—Methodologic challenges. *Biol. Blood Marrow Transplant.* **2011**, *17*, 1428–1435. [CrossRef] [PubMed]

9.   Clanton, N.R.; Klosky, J.L.; Li, C.; Jain, N.; Srivastava, D.K.; Mulrooney, D.; Zeltzer, L.; Stovall, M.; Robison, L.; Krull, K. Fatigue, vitality, sleep, and neurocognitive functioning in adult survivors of childhood cancer: A report from the childhood cancer survivor study. *Cancer* **2011**, *117*, 2559–2568. [CrossRef] [PubMed]

10.   Diller, L.; Chow, E.J.; Gurney, J.G.; Hudson, M.M.; Kadin-Lottick, N.S.; Kawashima, T.I.; Leisenring, W.M.; Meacham, L.R.; Mertens, A.C.; Mulrooney, D.A.; et al. Chronic disease in the childhood cancer survivor study cohort: A review of published findings. *J. Clin. Oncol.* **2009**, *27*, 2339–2355. [CrossRef] [PubMed]

11.   Feijen, E.A.M.; Font-Gonzalez, A.; van Dalen, E.C.; van der Pal, H.J.H.; Reulen, R.C.; Winter, D.L.; Kuehni, C.E.; Haupt, R.; Alessi, D.; Byrne, J.; et al. Late cardiac events after childhood cancer: Methodological aspects of the Pan-European study PanCareSurFup. *PLoS ONE* **2016**, *11*, e0162778. [CrossRef] [PubMed]

12.   Friedman, D.L.; Whitton, J.; Leisenring, W.; Mertens, A.C.; Hammond, S.; Stoval, M.; Donaldson, S.S.; Meadows, A.T.; Robison, L.L.; Neglia, J.P. Subsequent neoplasms in 5-year survivors of childhood cancer: The childhood cancer survivor study. *J. Natl. Cancer Inst.* **2010**, *102*, 1083–1095. [CrossRef] [PubMed]

13.   Gibson, T.M.; Robison, L.L. Impact of cancer therapy-related exposures on late mortality in childhood cancer survivors. *Chem. Res. Toxicol.* **2015**, *28*, 31–37. [CrossRef] [PubMed]

14.   Haupt, R.; Jankovic, M.; Hjorth, L.; Skinner, R. Late effects in childhood cancer survivors and survivorship issues. *Epidemiol. Prev.* **2013**, *37* (Suppl. 1), 1–296.

15.   Lipshultz, E.R.; Holt, G.E.; Ramasamy, R.; Yechieli, R.; Lipshultz, S.E. Fertility, cardiac, and orthopedic challenges in survivors of adult and childhood sarcoma. *Am. Soc. Clin. Oncol. Educ. Book* **2017**, *37*, 799–806. [CrossRef] [PubMed]

16.   Mulrooney, D.A.; Yeazel, M.W.; Kawashima, T.; Mertens, A.C.; Mitby, P.; Stovall, M.; Donaldson, S.S.; Green, D.M.; Sklar, C.A.; Robison, L.L.; et al. Cardiac outcomes in a cohort of adult survivors of childhood and adolescent cancer: Retrospective analysis of the Childhood Cancer Survivor Study cohort. *BMJ* **2009**, *339*, b4606. [CrossRef] [PubMed]

17.   Oeffinger, K.C.; Mertens, A.C.; Sklar, C.A.; Kawashima, T.; Hudson, M.M.; Meadows, A.T.; Friedman, D.L.; Marina, N.; Hobbie, W.; Kadan-Lottick, N.S.; et al. Childhood Cancer Survivor Study. Chronic health conditions in adult survivors of childhood cancer. *N. Engl. J. Med.* **2006**, *355*, 1572–1582. [CrossRef] [PubMed]

18.   Bhakta, N.; Liu, Q.; Yeo, F.; Baassiri, M.; Ehrhardt, M.J.; Srivastava, D.K.; Metzger, M.L.; Krasin, M.J.; Ness, K.K.; Hudson, M.M.; et al. Cumulative burden of cardiovascular morbidity in paediatric, adolescent, and young adult survivors of Hodgkin's lymphoma: An analysis from the St Jude Lifetime Cohort Study. *Lancet Oncol.* **2016**, *17*, 1325–1334. [CrossRef]

19.   Carneiro Teixeira, J.F.; Maia-Lemos, P.D.S.; Cypriano, M.D.S.; Pellegrini, P.L. Obesity in survivors of childhood cancer: A review. *Pediatr. Endocrinol. Rev.* **2017**, *15*, 33–39. [PubMed]

20.   Ligibel, J.A.; Alfano, C.M.; Courneya, K.S.; Demark-Wahnefried, W.; Burger, R.A.; Chlebowski, R.T.; Fabian, C.J.; Gucalp, A.; Hershman, D.L.; Hudson, M.M.; et al. American Society of Clinical Oncology position statement on obesity and cancer. *J. Clin. Oncol.* **2014**, *32*, 3568–3574. [CrossRef] [PubMed]

21.   Fernandez-Pineda, I.; Hudson, M.M.; Pappo, A.S.; Bishop, M.W.; Klosky, J.L.; Brinkman, T.M.; Srivastava, D.K.; Neel, M.D.; Rao, B.N.; Davidoff, A.M.; et al. Long-term functional outcomes and quality of life in adult survivors of childhood extremity sarcomas: A report from the St. Jude lifetime cohort study. *J. Cancer Surv.* **2017**, *11*, 1–12. [CrossRef] [PubMed]

22.   Gerber, L.H.; Hoffman, K.; Chaudhry, U.; Augustine, E.; Parks, R.; Bernad, M.; Mackall, C.; Steinberg, S.; Mansky, P. Functional outcomes and life satisfaction in long-term survivors of pediatric sarcomas. *Arch. Phys. Med. Rehabil.* **2006**, *87*, 1611–1617. [CrossRef] [PubMed]

23.   Ridola, V.; Fawaz, O.; Aubier, F.; Bergeron, C.; de Vathaire, F.; Orbach, D.; Gentet, J.C.; Schmitt, C.; Dufour, C.; Oberlin, O. Testicular function of survivors of childhood cancer: A comparative study between ifosfamide and cyclophosphamide-based regimens. *Eur. J. Cancer* **2009**, *45*, 814–818.

24.   Rose, S.R.; Danish, R.K.; Kearney, N.S.; Schreiber, R.E.; Lustig, R.H.; Burghen, G.A.; Hudson, M.M. ACTH deficiency in childhood cancer survivors. *Pediatr. Blood Cancer* **2005**, *45*, 808–813. [CrossRef] [PubMed]

25.   Siviero-Miachon, A.A.; Spinola-Castro, A.M.; Guerra-Junior, G. Detection of metabolic syndrome features among childhood cancer survivors: A target to prevent disease. *Vasc. Health Risk Manag.* **2008**, *4*, 825–836. [PubMed]

26. Skinner, R.; Mulder, R.L.; Kremer, L.C.; Hudson, M.M.; Constine, L.S.; Bardi, E.; Boekhout, A.; Borgmann-Staudt, A.; Brown, M.C.; Cohn, R.; et al. Recommendations for gonadotoxicity surveillance in male childhood, adolescent, and young adult cancer survivors: A report from the International Late Effects of Childhood Cancer Guideline Harmonization Group in collaboration with the PanCareSurFup Consortium. *Lancet Oncol.* **2017**, *18*, e75–e90.

27. Massimino, M.; Gandola, L.; Mattavelli, F.; Pizzi, N.; Seregni, E.; Pallotti, F.; Spreafico, F.; Marchianò, A.; Terenziani, M.; Cefalo, G.; et al. Radiation-induced thyroid changes: A retrospective and a prospective view. *Eur. J. Cancer* **2009**, *45*, 2546–2551. [CrossRef] [PubMed]

28. Hartman, A.; te Winkel, M.L.; van Beek, R.D.; de Muinck Keizer-Schrama, S.M.P.F.; Kemper, H.C.G.; Hop, W.C.J.; van den Heuvel-Eibrink, M.M.; Pieters, R. A randomized trial investigating an exercise program to prevent reduction of bone mineral density and impairment of motor performance during treatment for childhood acute lymphoblastic leukemia. *Pediatr. Blood Cancer* **2009**, *53*, 64–71. [CrossRef] [PubMed]

29. Hudson, M.M.; Mertens, A.C.; Yasui, Y.; Hobbie, W.; Chen, H.; Gurney, J.G.; Yeazel, M.; Recklitis, C.J.; Marina, N.; Robison, L.R.; et al. Health status of adult long-term survivors of childhood cancer: A report from the childhood cancer survivor study. *JAMA* **2003**, *290*, 1583–1592. [CrossRef] [PubMed]

30. Hudson, M.M.; Ness, K.K.; Gurney, J.G.; Mulrooney, D.A.; Chemaitilly, W.; Krull, K.R.; Green, D.M.; Armstrong, G.T.; Nottage, K.A.; Jones, K.E.; et al. Clinical ascertainment of health outcomes among adults treated for childhood cancer. *JAMA* **2013**, *309*, 2371–2381. [CrossRef] [PubMed]

31. Skinner, R. Nephrotoxicity—What do we know and what don't we know? *J. Pediatr. Hematol. Oncol.* **2011**, *33*, 128–134. [CrossRef] [PubMed]

32. Sklar, C.A.; Mertens, A.C.; Mitby, P.; Whitton, J.; Stovall, M.; Kasper, C.; Mulder, J.; Green, D.; Nicholson, H.S.; Yasui, Y.; et al. Premature menopause in survivors of childhood cancer: A report from the childhood cancer survivor study. *J. Natl. Cancer Inst.* **2006**, *98*, 890–896. [CrossRef] [PubMed]

33. Interiano, R.B.; Kaste, S.C.; Li, C.; Srivastava, D.K.; Rao, B.N.; Warner, W.C.Jr.; Green, D.M.; Krasin, M.J.; Robison, L.L.; Davidoff, A.M.; Hudson, M.M.; et al. Associations between treatment, scoliosis, pulmonary function, and physical performance in long-term survivors of sarcoma. *J. Cancer Surv.* **2017**, *11*. [CrossRef] [PubMed]

34. Ness, K.K.; Armstrong, G.T.; Kundu, M.; Wilson, C.L.; Tchkonia, T.; Kirkland, J.L. Frailty in childhood cancer survivors. *Cancer* **2015**, *121*, 1540–1547. [CrossRef] [PubMed]

35. Ness, K.K.; Krull, K.R.; Jones, K.E.; Mulrooney, D.A.; Armstrong, G.T.; Green, D.M.; Chemaitilly, W.; Smith, W.A.; Wilson, C.L.; Sklar, C.A.; et al. Physiologic frailty as a sign of accelerated aging among adult survivors of childhood cancer: A report from the St Jude Lifetime Cohort Study. *J. Clin. Oncol.* **2013**, *31*, 4496–4503. [CrossRef] [PubMed]

36. Winther, J.F.; Kenborg, L.; Byrne, J.; Hjorth, L.; Kaatsch, P.; Kremer, L.C.; Kuehni, C.E.; Auquier, P.; Michel, G.; de Vathaire, F.; et al. Childhood cancer survivor cohorts in Europe. *Acta Oncol.* **2015**, *54*, 655–668. [CrossRef] [PubMed]

37. Wilson, C.L.; Chemaitilly, W.; Jones, K.E.; Kaste, S.C.; Srivastava, D.K.; Ojha, R.P.; Yasui, Y.; Pui, C.-H.; Robison, L.L.; Hudson, M.M.; et al. Modifiable factors associated with aging phenotypes among adult survivors of childhood acute lymphoblastic leukemia. *J. Clin. Oncol.* **2016**, *34*, 2509–2515. [CrossRef] [PubMed]

38. Schmitz, K.H.; Courneya, K.S.; Matthews, C.; Demark-Wahnefried, W.; Galvão, D.A.; Pinto, B.M.; Irwin, M.L.; Wolin, K.Y.; Segal, R.J.; Lucia, A.; et al. American College of Sports Medicine roundtable on exercise guidelines for cancer survivors. *Med. Sci. Sports Exerc.* **2010**, *42*, 1409–1426. [CrossRef] [PubMed]

39. Braam, K.I.; van der Torre, P.; Takken, T.; Veening, M.A.; van Dulmen-den Broeder, E.; Kaspers, G.J.L. Physical exercise training interventions for children and young adults during and after treatment for childhood cancer. *Cochrane Database Syst. Rev.* **2013**, *4*. [CrossRef]

40. Huang, T.-T.; Ness, K.K. Exercise interventions in children with cancer: A review. *Int. J. Pediatr.* **2011**, 1–11. [CrossRef]

41. Deisenroth, A.; Söntgerath, R.; Schuster, A.J.; von Busch, C.; Huber, G.; Eckert, K.; Kulozik, A.E.; Wiskemann, J. Muscle strength and quality of life in patients with childhood cancer at early phase of primary treatment. *Pediatr. Hematol. Oncol.* **2016**, *33*, 393–407. [CrossRef] [PubMed]

42. Esbenshade, A.J.; Friedman, D.L.; Smith, W.A.; Jeha, S.; Pui, C.H.; Robison, L.L.; Ness, K.K. Feasibility and initial effectiveness of home exercise during maintenance therapy for childhood acute lymphoblastic leukemia. *Pediatr. Phys. Ther.* **2014**, *26*, 301–307. [CrossRef] [PubMed]
43. Keats, M.R.; Culos-Reed, S.N. A community-based physical activity program for adolescents with cancer (project TREK): Program feasibility and preliminary findings. *J. Pediatr. Hematol./Oncol.* **2008**, *30*, 272–280. [CrossRef] [PubMed]
44. Rueegg, C.S.; Michel, G.; Wengenroth, L.; von der Weid, N.X.; Bergstraesser, E.; Kuehni, C.E. Physical performance limitations in adolescent and adult survivors of childhood cancer and their siblings. *PLoS ONE* **2012**, *7*, e47944. [CrossRef] [PubMed]
45. Wurz, A.; Brunet, J. The effects of physical activity on health and quality of life in adolescent cancer survivors: A systematic review. *JMIR Cancer* **2016**, *2*, e6. [CrossRef] [PubMed]
46. Zhang, F.F.; Kelly, M.J.; Aviva, M. Early nutrition and physical activity interventions in childhood cancer survivors. *Curr. Obes. Rep.* **2017**, *6*, 168–177. [CrossRef] [PubMed]
47. Zhang, F.F.; Meagher, S.; Scheurer, M.; Folta, S.; Finnan, E.; Criss, K.; Economos, C.; Dreyer, Z.; Kelly, M. Developing a web-based weight management program for childhood cancer survivors: Rationale and methods. *JMIR Res. Protoc.* **2016**, *5*, e214. [CrossRef] [PubMed]
48. Zhang, F.F.; Parsons, S.K. Obesity in childhood cancer survivors: Call for early weight management. *Adv. Nutr.* **2015**, *6*, 611–619. [CrossRef] [PubMed]
49. Fairey, A.S.; Courneya, K.S.; Field, C.J.; Mackey, J.R. Physical exercise and immune system function in cancer survivors: A comprehensive review and future direction. *Cancer* **2002**, *94*, 539–551. [CrossRef] [PubMed]
50. Malina, R.M.; Bouchard, C.; Bar-Or, O. *Growth, Maturation, and Physical Activity*, 2nd ed.; Human Kinetics: Champaign, IL, USA, 2004; pp. 3–18.
51. Li, T.; Wei, S.; Shi, Y.; Pang, S.; Qin, Q.; Yin, J.; Deng, Y.; Chen, Q.; Wei, S.; Nie, S.; et al. The dose-response effect of physical activity on cancer mortality: Findings from 71 prospective cohort studies. *Br. J. Sports Med.* **2016**, *50*, 339. [CrossRef] [PubMed]
52. Hjorth, L.; Haupt, R.; Skinner, R.; Grabow, D.; Byrne, J.; Karner, S.; Levitt, G.; Michel, G.; van Der Pal, H.; Bárdi, E.; et al. Survivorship after childhood cancer: PanCare: A European network to promote optimal long-term care. *Eur. J. Cancer* **2015**, *1*, 1203–1211. [CrossRef] [PubMed]
53. Wallace, W.H.; Blacklay, A.; Eiser, C.; Davies, H.; Hawkins, M.; Levitt, G.A.; Jenney, M.E.M. Regular review: Developing strategies for long term follow up of survivors of childhood cancer. *BMJ* **2001**, *323*, 271–274. [CrossRef] [PubMed]
54. American Academy of Pediatrics Section on Hematology/Oncology, Children's Oncology Group Long-Term Follow-Up Care for Pediatric Cancer Survivors. *Pediatrics* **2009**, *123*, 906–915. [CrossRef]
55. Castellino, S.M.; Ullrich, N.J.; Whelen, M.J.; Lange, B.J. Developing interventions for cancer-related cognitive dysfunction in childhood cancer survivors. *J. Natl. Cancer Inst.* **2014**, *106*, 1–16. [CrossRef] [PubMed]
56. Langeveld, N.E.; Grootenhuis, M.A.; Voûte, P.A.; de Haan, R.J.; van den Bos, C. Quality of life, self-esteem and worries in young adult survivors of childhood cancer. *Psychooncology* **2004**, *13*, 867–881. [CrossRef] [PubMed]
57. Huang, I.-C.; Brinkman, T.M.; Armstrong, G.T.; Leisenring, W.; Robison, L.L.; Krull, K.R. Emotional distress impacts quality of life evaluation: A report from the Childhood Cancer Survivor Study. *J. Cancer Surv.* **2017**, *11*, 309–319. [CrossRef] [PubMed]
58. Varni, J.W.; Katz, E.R.; Seid, M.; Quiggins, D.J.L.; Friedman-Bender, A. The pediatric cancer quality of life inventory-32 (PCQL-32). *Cancer* **1998**, *82*, 1184–1196. [CrossRef]
59. The Children's Oncology Group. Long-Term Follow-Up Guidelines for Survivors of Childhood, Adolescent, and Young Adult Cancers. Available online: http://www.survivorshipguidelines.org/ (accessed on 20 December 2017).
60. Lohman, T.G.; Roche, A.F.; Martorell, R. (Eds.) *Anthropometric Standardization Reference Manual*; Human Kinetics; Information Systems Division, Naional Agricultural Library: Champaign, IL, USA, 1988.
61. Stewart, A.; Marfell-Jones, M. *International Standards for Anthropometric Assessment*; International Society for the Advancement of Kinanthropometry: Lower Hutt, New Zealand, 2011.
62. Roche, A.F.; Malina, R.M. *Manual of Physical Status and Performance in Childhood*; Plenum Press: New York, NY, USA, 1983; p. 1.

63. Bachrach, L.K.; Sills, I.N. Clinical report-bone densitometry in children and adolescents. *Pediatrics* **2011**, *127*, 189–194. [CrossRef] [PubMed]

64. Cox, C.l.; Zuh, L.; Ojha, R.P.; Steen, B.D.; Ogg, S.; Robison, L.L.; Hudson, M.M. Factors supporting cardiomyopathy screening among at-risk adult survivors of pediatric malignancies. *Support Care Cancer* **2017**, *25*, 1307–1316. [CrossRef] [PubMed]

65. Golden, E.; Beach, B.; Hastings, C. The pediatrician and medical care of the child with cancer. *Pediatr. Clin. N. Am.* **2002**, *49*, 1319–1338. [CrossRef]

66. Stefani, L.; Pedrizzetti, G.; Galanti, G. Clinical application of 2D speckle tracking strain for assessing cardio-toxicity in oncology. *J. Funct. Morphol. Kinesiol.* **2016**, *1*, 343–354. [CrossRef]

67. Voigt, J.U.; Pedrizzetti, G.; Lysyansky, P.; Marwick, T.M.; Houle, H.; Baumann, R.; Pedri, S.; Ito, Y.; Abe, Y.; Metz, S.; et al. Definitions for a common standard for 2D Speckle tracking echocardiography: Consensus document of the EACVI/ASE/industry task force to standardize deformation imaging. *Eur. Heart J. Cardiovasc. Imaging* **2015**, *16*, 1–11. [CrossRef] [PubMed]

68. Yu, A.F.; Raikhelkar, J.; Zabor, E.C.; Tonorezos, E.S.; Moskowitz, C.S.; Adsuar, R.; Mara, E.; Huie, K.; Oeffinger, K.C.; Steingart, R.M.; et al. Two-dimensional speckle tracking echocardiography detects subclinical left ventricular systolic dysfunction among adult survivors of childhood, adolescent, and young adult cancer. *Cancer Biomed. Res. Int.* **2016**. [CrossRef] [PubMed]

69. Leger, L. Aerobic performance. In *Measurement in Pediatric Exercise Science*; Dougherty, D., Ed.; Human Kinetics: Champaign, IL, USA, 1996; pp. 183–223.

70. Borg, G.; Hassmen, P.; Whipp, B.J. Perceived exertion in relation to heart rate and blood lactate 12 during and arm and leg exercise. *Eur. J. Appl. Physiol.* **1985**, *65*, 679–685.

71. Bayley, N. Bayley scales of infant and toddler development: Administration manual. In *Harcourt Assessment*; Pearson: San Antonio, TX, USA, 2006.

72. Naumann, F.L.; Hunt, M.; Ali, D.; Wakefield, C.E.; Moultrie, K.; Cohn, R.J. Assessment of fundamental motor skills in childhood cancer patients. *Pediatr. Blood Cancer* **2015**, *62*, 2211–2215. [CrossRef] [PubMed]

73. Moultrie, K.; Cohn, R.J. Assessment of gross motor skills and phenotype profile in children 9-11 years of age in survivors of acute lymphoblastic leukemia. *Pediatr. Blood Cancer* **2015**, *1*, 46–52. [CrossRef]

74. Perry, J.; Davids, J.R. Gait analysis: Normal and pathological function. *J. Pediatr. Orthop.* **1992**, *126*, 815. [CrossRef]

75. U.S. Department of Health and Human Services. *Physical Activity Guidelines for Americans*; Department of Health and Human Services: Washington, DC, USA, 2008.

76. McNeely, M.L.; Peddle, C.J.; Parliament, M.; Courneya, K.S. Cancer rehabilitation: Recommendations for integrating exercise programming in a clinical setting. *Curr. Cancer Ther. Rev.* **2006**, *2*, 251–260. [CrossRef]

77. Malina, R.M. Movement proficiency in childhood: Implications for physical activity and youth sport. *Kinesiol. Slov.* **2012**, *18*, 19–34.

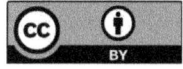

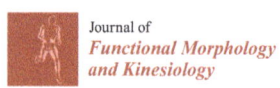

Journal of
Functional Morphology and Kinesiology

Protocol

Feasibility Study of the Secondary Level Active School Flag Programme: Study Protocol

Kwok W Ng [1,2,*], Fiona McHale [1], Karen Cotter [3], Donal O'Shea [4] and Catherine Woods [1]

[1]   Department of Physical Education and Sport Sciences; Centre of Physical Activity and Health Research; Health Research Institute, University of Limerick, V94 T9PX Limerick, Ireland; fiona.mchale@ul.ie (F.M.); catherine.woods@ul.ie (C.W.)

[2]   School of Educational Sciences and Psychology, University of Eastern Finland, 80101 Joensuu, Finland

[3]   Active Schools Flag, Mayo Education Centre, F23 HX48 Castlebar, Ireland; karen@activeschoolflag.ie

[4]   St. Vincent's University Hospital, University College Dublin, D04 T6F4 Dublin, Ireland; info@dosheaendo.ie

*   Correspondence: kwok.ng@ul.ie or kwok.ng@uef.fi; Tel.: +358-50-472-4051

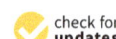

Received: 27 February 2019; Accepted: 19 March 2019; Published: 26 March 2019

Abstract: Taking part in regular physical activity (PA) is important for young adolescents to maintain physical, social and mental health. Schools are vibrant settings for health promotion and the complexity of driving a whole-school approach to PA has not been tested in the Irish school context. The feasibility of the pilot programme of the Department of Education and Skills second level Active School Flag (SLASF) is needed. SLASF is a two year process that consists of the Active School Flag (ASF) certificate programme (year 1) and the ASF flag programme (year 2). This protocol paper is specific to the first year certificate process. Three schools around Ireland were recruited as pilot schools to carry out the year-long SLASF programme with 17 planned actions involving the entire school. Students in the transition year programme have a particular role in the promotion of PA in SLASF. Data collection consists of physical measures, accelerometers, survey data and interviews at the beginning and the end of the academic year. The primary focus on the feasibility of the programme is through process evaluation tools and fidelity checks consisting of implementation of the SLASF programme through whole-school surveys, focus group discussions of key stakeholder groups, as well as one-to-one interviews with a member of management at each school and the SLASF coordinator of the school. Secondary outcomes include PA levels and its social cognitive theories based correlates through physical health measures, surveys carried out pre- and post-intervention, as well as focus group discussions of the students. The results of this study are needed to improve the development of the SLASF through a predetermined stopping criteria and inclusion into systems thinking approaches such as the Healthy Ireland Demonstration Project.

Keywords: physical activity; adolescent; health promotion; activePal; intervention

---

1. Introduction

There are multiple reasons—physical, psychological, social, environmental—health for adolescents to take part in regular physical activity (PA). However, adolescence forms a highly volatile stage in life where transitional periods can influence behaviour [1] and is a critical time for PA participation where habits—good or bad—developed, later persist into adulthood [2]. Despite the evidence of health benefits from PA, a clear reduction in PA levels is apparent alongside increasing age in adolescence. Data from the Children's Sport Participation and Physical Activity (CSPPA) study highlighted a decline in meeting the PA guidelines, at least 60 min of moderate-to-vigorous (MVPA) per day, from 18% among 12y olds (first year of second level education in Ireland) to 6% among 18y olds (last year of second level education in Ireland) [3]. Similarly, a systematic review and pooled analysis indicated that PA levels decline by a mean of 7% per year over this period [4,5]. By the age of 15y, on average, across 42 countries in the Health Behaviour in School-aged Children study, only 11% of girls and 21% of boys self-reported sufficient MVPA levels [6]. Global PA decline throughout adolescence, across a range of measurement units, appears as high as 60–70% [4]. Action is needed to reduce the drop in PA levels.

Actions that target the drop in PA levels can include interventions at the individual, community and within policy [7]. Although policy interventions may provide the best return on investment [8], creating such changes requires a strong evidence base that interventions targeting the behaviours actually works. At the individual level, interventions that were designed to increase school-based PA levels have yet to demonstrate its effectiveness [8]. In particular, multi-component PA interventions have yet to demonstrate improvements in overall MVPA [9]. However, at the community level, school-based PA programmes have demonstrated some positive effect on overall PA levels [10].

1.1. Whole-School Approaches to Physical Activity Promotion

Successfully run school-based PA programmes includes quality physical education, physical activities before-, during- and after-school, at the school grounds, as well as activities based in the local community [11]. Haapala and colleagues [11] suggested that recess time activities before, during and after school are opportune moments to promote PA. Similarly, a study based on a 12 week walking intervention among girls who took part before-school and during recess times increased the time in light intensity PA by 10 min but differences in MVPA were not statistically significant when compared to the intervention group [12]. Some recent studies have investigated the role of peers in boosting PA levels. For example, peer leaders (15–16y olds) slightly older than the target group (13–15y olds) encouraged after-school activities. By the end of the 7-week after-school intervention, there was a statistically significant increase of three minutes of daily MVPA [13]. Same-aged peers were also effective in promoting six minutes of daily MVPA through diffusion messages among girls during the entire school day [14]. Statistically significant changes on PA levels were found for those identified as low active at baseline in an intervention that focused on increasing step count in both boys and girls [15]. Few school-based programmes managed to succeed in increasing boys' PA levels for school-based interventions through a peer-led model [16,17]. Programmes with in-class activities that promote PA by the class teachers are another way to increase PA levels [18]. The latter activities requires a whole-school approach towards PA promotion and in Ireland, this is known as the Active School Flag (ASF) [19].

The ASF (www.activeschoolflag.ie) is a Department of Education and Skills (DES) initiative supported by Healthy Ireland. It takes a 'whole-school approach' and requires all members of the school community to work together to strengthen the delivery of the physical education programme and to promote PA throughout the school in a fun and inclusive manner. It emphasises quality PE, co-curricular PA as well as partnerships with students, parents and the wider community. In 2018, 29% ($N = 1329$) of primary schools in Ireland had achieved ASF status. Some have the need for renewal, thus at the time of print, 722 primary schools currently have possession of an Active Flag. The journey towards achieving this status begins with self-evaluation in the areas of (i) physical education (ii) PA and (iii) partnerships. Following this, schools are expected to devise a strategic plan and implement changes to help improve the quality of PE, provide additional opportunities for PA and support additional involvement with the wider community. Lastly, the school has to provide a week-long focus on PA in an Active School Week.

The ASF is well-established as a primary school initiative but has yet to be developed for the secondary level education sector. A generic model has been tried among secondary level schools, although it did not achieve the same effect because the uptake of secondary level schools is below 5%. The most notable differences were the lack of whole-school engagement in the secondary level schools. Feedback from those experiences suggested that the generic ASF in secondary level was viewed as a physical education programme as opposed to a whole-school initiative. Furthermore, there are structural differences between primary and secondary level schools, thus a direct translation of the primary ASF to the secondary level setting would be specious. Some examples of differences include; in primary schools, a single teacher generally remains with the same class throughout the entire day, whereas at secondary level schools, students are taught by multiple teachers. In the secondary level schools, many schools do not have a compulsory timetabled physical education in accordance with DES recommendations (i.e., a double timetabled period for all students every week). Secondary level schools tend to be larger and cater for more students than primary schools, yet facilities for promoting PA can be limiting. Peer influences tend to be stronger at secondary level education [20] and students will often choose to socialise with their friends and be sedentary rather than take part in PA [21]. In primary schools, all teachers are encouraged to take part in continuous professional development (CPD) as part of their classroom responsibility in the areas of physical education and PA. Class teachers in secondary level schools tend to be specialists in their subject area and may not have the confidence or competence to create active breaks in the classroom [22].

In the majority of Irish secondary level schools, there is the 'Transition Year' (TY) period, whereby it is non- examinable and students may go on to try out activities beyond the normal school curriculum [23]. The aims of TY are to "increase social awareness and social competence with 'education through experience of adult and working life' as a basis for personal development and maturity" [24]. TY programmes can cover various aspects of personal development, including visits to hospitals to learn about health behaviours [25], as well as taking part in other science programmes [26]. Many TY based programmes seek to develop youth leadership skills (i.e., Gaisce the President's Award, Young Social Innovators, Gaelic Athletic Association (GAA) future leaders, etc.).

1.2. Theoretical Background to the Study

The theoretical premise of this feasibility study is underpinned by social cognitive theories [27] These theories are the most cited for health behaviour change interventions [28]. In these theories, there is a triad relationship between personal and environmental factors with behaviours being explored through individual level factors such as self-efficacy, stages of readiness for behavioural change and school related autonomy. In self-efficacy theory [29] there are four sources; mastery accomplishments, vicarious experiences, verbal persuasion and physiology are strong predictors of behaviour. Novice learners, such as students in TY, tend to have low confidence to promote PA at the beginning of the year [30]. When schools express their interest to be an SLASF school, a resource pack (see methods section) would support these students to improve the self-efficacy (opportunities for mastery accomplishments), create timetabled meetings with the purpose to focus on the SLASF (opportunities for vicarious experiences) and regular contact with others who are also carrying out the SLASF (opportunities for verbal persuasions), the sources of self-efficacy may create a better suited environment for promoting PA.

Being autonomous in making decisions is known to be directly related to intrinsic motivations towards a behaviour [31]. However, in the school context, students may feel their overall autonomy is restricted to the bounds of the school. As a result, some students may find the school environment something that they can thrive in, whereas others may feel the environment restricts individual choices. The autonomy supportive environment is as important as having autonomy among school-aged children because it can lead to greater levels of PA outside of the school context [32]. Factors that may influence the autonomy or autonomy support can include the perception of school academic performance and the way teachers and peers support academic performance [33], perceptions of ability to make decisions in the school [34] and feelings of belonging in the school [35]. Furthermore, it has been reported that individual well-being is associated with individual's sense of autonomy [36], therefore studies may need to consider the mediating factors of student well-being.

The levels of readiness for taking part in regular PA would vary vastly among the students throughout the school. According to the transtheoretical model [37] individuals are at different stages of their intention for behavioural change. Progression between the five noted stages include pre-contemplation (not ready), contemplation (getting ready), preparation (ready), action and maintenance. According to the model, the factors that influence moving between these stages consist of biopsychosocial factors, including self-efficacy, own and socially supported decisions and going through the process of change [38]. Through awareness of the stages of change among the target population, there is a greater understanding of how to create targeted interventions for the promotion of PA.

1.3. Measures of Feasibility

The SLASF programme is in its pilot phase as part of a larger systems based Healthy Ireland Demonstration Project. It is also a feasibility study, because we aim to investigate whether it is suitable in secondary level schools and if so, how to do that [39]. According to Bowen and colleagues [40], designing feasibility studies can have eight areas of focus; acceptability, demand, implementation, practicality, adaptation, integration, expansion and limited efficacy. Although the SLASF is a non-clinical study, the feasibility study is useful to provide an indicator for stopping, revisions or continuing for a scaling up a randomised control trial [41]. Moreover, the predefined rules need to be put in place prior to the analysis to prevent uncontrollable biases [42]. In Table 1, Bowen and colleagues' areas of foci for this feasibility study are broken down into the areas which this study researches and stopping criteria.

Table 1. Areas of focus for feasibility studies with measures and stopping criteria.

Focus	Measures	Stopping Criteria
Acceptability	Pragmatic survey instrument on suitability, satisfying and attractiveness for SLASF in schools for the TY and the whole-school at the end of the year.	When less than half the school students and TY consider SLASF to be suitable, satisfying or attractive to them.
	Focus group and interviews to describe the process of satisfaction of the programme, fit into the school's culture and the positive and negative effect on the school.	When interviews describe strong statements that have a negative impact on the school's culture or too much dissatisfaction to the programme.
Demand	PA audit of sections of the school.	No improvement over the academic year.
	Attendance list at the specific activities	Unsustainable numbers in attendance.
	Survey instrument based on readiness for PA behaviours.	Over half of students increased their readiness if they can.
	Focus groups based on the TY engagement in the SLASF process.	Discussions confirm low attendance rates and lack of demand for activities.
Implementation	Action Logs from the logbook.	Over half actions left incomplete
	Focus groups on implementation ease	Discussions where respondents report too many challenges preventing implementation
	Staff interviews	Data that suggests lack of resources to implement the programme and failures to execute the actions.
Practicality	Action plans for promotion of PA	If action plans could not be drawn up by the specified time frame
Adaptation	Registrations at events carried out as part of the action plan	Substantial decrease in participation over a 6 week period
Integration	Pre- and post-test results on PA opportunities and its participation	No increased opportunities since the beginning of the programme.
	Interviews with management about costs to organization and school policies	Descriptions whereby the costs are not sustainable. Indicators that there is a lack of staff
Expansion	Interviews of management	Descriptions of the uniqueness of the programme to the school and difficulties to roll out to other schools.
Limited Efficacy	Pre- and post-test results from the comprehensive surveys	Reduction in main outcome variables over the course of the year that is greater than the difference between each year cohort at the baseline measurements
	ASF logbook entries	Notes that report barriers to completing actions that are not manageable
	PA audit	Low level of usage when compared with the beginning of the year

1.4. Purpose of the Study

The primary objective for this study is to see if the SLASF certificate is an acceptable programme in secondary level Irish schools. The secondary objectives are to see how feasible it is to operationalise the components needed for testing a year-long intervention. These include collecting accelerometer and physical health measures of students in the schools, completion of survey questions for pre- and post-intervention evaluation and investigate areas for improvement from a pilot study to scale-up intervention programme.

2. Methods and Design

2.1. Setting

Eligible schools include secondary level schools in the Republic of Ireland that have not previously applied for the SLASF. Special educational needs schools or schools without a range of students from each year group are excluded. The feasibility study will be conducted in three secondary level schools, covering the demographics of a girls only school, a mixed school with designated 'Delivering Equality of Opportunity in Schools' (DEIS) status and a mixed mainstream school. A DEIS school is part of the Department of Education and Skill's action plan for educational inclusion to address disadvantaged education.

2.2. Recruitment

2.2.1. School Recruitment

The SLASF programme is a comprehensive programme and employs a whole school approach. As an intervention programme, schools were invited to take part if they are not currently in the process of obtaining the Active School Flag. The normal process of the SLASF recruitment is for schools to make an application but this was suspended to allow time to develop the new model. Schools that were interested in carrying out the feasibility study contacted the Active Schools office and requested to pilot the second level programme. There were three schools that responded and accepted because they each have a strong well-being structure in place in their schools. This is a feasibility study with secondary outcomes on efficacy hence matched control schools (one girls only, one mixed and one mixed DEIS school) were recruited to take part in the survey component of the study. No reserve list was formed for this cohort but engagement of all three schools throughout the year to follow the feasibility and evaluate the SLASF process.

2.2.2. Student Recruitment

In the participating schools, there are two levels of student engagement—basic and comprehensive. Although all students are exposed to the same SLASF programme, those engaged in the SLASF Basic are required to complete less data collection measures than those in the SLASF Comprehensive. The whole school is involved in the SLASF Basic and a random class from each year group is selected to take part in the SLASF Comprehensive. Classes are known as mixed ability tutor groups. Students obtain their consent to take part in the study. Even though there may be some students who do not obtain consent or would not like to withdraw from the comprehensive aspect of the study, there is no likely reason for them to influence the feasibility of the study.

The SLASF initiative is structured to fit into the TY framework providing real and meaningful opportunities for student voice and youth leadership. A TY class would be nominated by the school as the SLASF TY class. This TY class attends classes in relation to SLASF tasks including youth leadership, mentoring and PA promotion.

2.3. Consent

All students are given information letters for their parents. The information stated the purpose of the study as well as components of the study that would involve their child. Also, the letter invites the parents to speak to their children about the study and there are contact details to the research team to answer questions the parents may have. Because of population bias from active consent, passive consent was used for all students in the basic part of the programme. The school manages the returned forms of withdrawal. This is because it is part of the whole-school process and as a feasibility of programme, schools need to be aware of how to handle withdrawal from the programme. The online survey requests the students to give their assent (if under the age of 16) or consent (if over the age of 16).

Students assigned to the comprehensive study, receive the same information sheets as the basic programme but in addition, information about the other measures that are included as part of the feasibility and process evaluation. Parents are asked to give opt in consent due to the nature of data collection (i.e., use of accelerometers). As part of Irish law, students over the age of 16 can give their own consent to take part in the study. All students were asked to opt in to be included in video recordings of interviews.

2.4. Allocation Strategy

There was no allocation strategy used to select the schools. As a feasibility study, it was important to test the SLASF in various contexts. Three contexts were chosen; a DEIS school, a girls only school and a mixed school. All schools are considered to be large in size and this would test out the possible whole-school approach.

2.5. Active School Flag Intervention

The SLASF feasibility model is co-designed by a SLASF steering group and staff, researchers of the University of Limerick and feedback from the three lead schools. The SLASF process is designed to be peer-led by a TY SLASF class, who will have the support of an SLASF coordinator, SLASF committee members, school staff and school management. The initiative challenges peers to find ways to encourage more students in their school to engage in school-based PA opportunities (year 1—SLASF certificate) and community-based PA opportunities (year 2—SLASF flag). During year 1 (Active School Flag certificate) the focus is on increasing participation in school-based PA opportunities. Year 2 (Active School Flag) is focused on community-based activities.

Previously the SLASF was viewed as a physical education initiative. In order to generate greater whole-school engagement, the SLASF tasks are formatted to draw support for the SLASF TY team from school management and teachers across a variety of different subjects. The new format of the SLASF process complements two current key educational initiatives: The Well-Being Framework by the Irish National Council for Curriculum and Assessment, the School Self-Evaluation process by the Department of Education and Skills and a new initiative presently at draft stage: The Parent and Student Charter also by the Department of Education and Skills. Students working towards Gaisce the President's Award can use their SLASF work to fulfil their Community or Personal Skill challenge requirement. Another benefit of SLASF is that it will link schools with the current national Healthy Ireland PA programmes and national youth charity events including:

- Get Ireland Walking—www.getirelandwalking.ie
- Parkrun—www.parkrun.ie
- Get Ireland Swimming—www.swimireland.ie/get-swimming
- Swim for a Mile Challenge—www.swimireland.ie/get-swimming/swim-for-a-mile
- Darkness into Light—www.darknessintolight.ie
- Cycle Against Suicide—www.cycleagainstsuicide.com

The SLASF programme is a whole-school approach to increase PA opportunities and generate opportunities for student voice and youth leadership. Currently, there are two levels. The first level is a certificate. This is open to all secondary level schools. It can serve as a good link from primary schools to continue on the ethos of active schools and allow a school to consider whether to take the next step or not. Moreover, SLASF is a DES (Department of Education and Skills) initiative and it can only be awarded to schools that adhere to physical education timetable recommendations that is, a double timetabled period of physical education for all year groups. This provision is not in place in a large number of secondary level schools, thus heretofore excluding them from the SLASF process. The introduction of the certificate level, without eligibility criteria, opens the SLASF process to all interested post primary schools. If the SLASF certificate proves beneficial it may encourage them to revisit their timetable policy.

Achievement of the flag is a whole school process, meaning that management, staff and students all play a role in the programme. There is a requirement for website updates and an online presence. In order to achieve the SLASF Certificate a number of tasks must be completed during year 1. These include: (1) a staff slideshow, (2) an SLASF team slideshow, (3) class time slideshow (4) SLASF training day, (5) an SLASF awareness week (towards the beginning of the year), (6) website showcase, (7) SLASF whole school questionnaire, (8) SLASF launch event, (9) SLASF action plan, (10) 'Did You Know?' campaign, (11) PA module as part of Social, personal and health education (SPHE) subject for junior cycle students, (12) Active School WALKWAY, (13) Community Mapping of extra curriculum activities, (14) Community Event, (15) Active School Week, (16) SLASF accreditation visit and (17) school PA space audits (Figure 1).

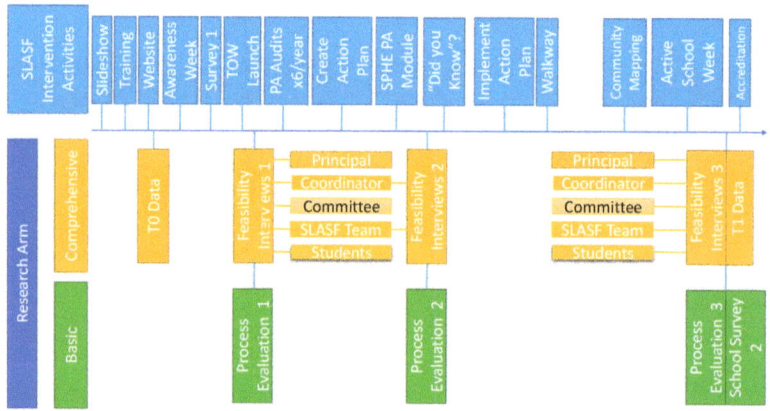

Figure 1. Second Level Active School Flag (SLASF) Intervention and Research Components Timeline.

All 17 activities are scheduled throughout the school year including a combination of staff and students as the main actors in this process. The SLASF TY class should take leadership guided and supported by the SLASF coordinator and committee on the programme. A key part of the process is that the SLASF coordinator has timetable provision allocated to two class periods per week to carry out work with the TY class. The committee includes staff representatives from the school, including one from management, an SLASF coordinator, two other staff who work on the well-being curriculum to include SPHE, Civic, Social, Political Education (CSPE) and Physical Education teachers, as well as four youth leaders. Structure of different actors in the process can be viewed in Figure 2.

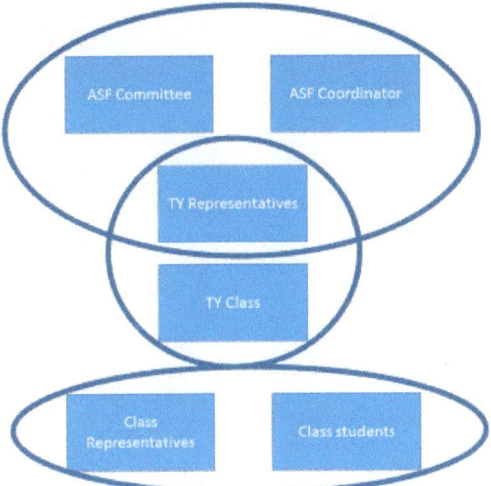

Figure 2. Actors of the Second Level Active school Flag.

Schools wishing to work towards the second level of the SLASF process, the Active School Flag, must have completed the certificate level and be able to confirm that they timetable physical education in accordance with DES recommendations.

At the student level, there are three levels of involvement. There is the SLASF team, which is comprised of the SLASF TY programme group. There are four SLASF youth leaders who represent the team at the school committee level. To be a youth leader, the SLASF team member needs to apply for the position through an application process that is evaluated by the staff members of the SLASF committee. The youth leaders end up representing the student voice at the SLASF committee and have the responsibility of presenting the SLASF action plan and the SLASF end of year review to the school Principal. The third student level is the SLASF class representatives. There are two in every class in the school and students can also apply for this position through an application form. The selection will be made by the class tutor in consultation with the SLASF coordinator.

2.5.1. TY Leader Role

The TY leader role is responsible for planning, promoting and implementing the SLASF initiatives and events throughout the school year. Based on self-efficacy theory [29], TY leaders are a closer connection to the students in the schools than teachers, thus strengthen vicarious experiences. Moreover, social support and leadership from the TYs can reinforce the basic premise of proactive behaviour change [43]. The SLASF team can be identified by being given pins to wear on their uniform. Moreover, part of the time spent on SLASF activities can be used as part of a time bank for other volunteering programmes, such as, Gaisce the President's Award. The selected SLASF youth leaders will receive their own distinct pins to wear on the uniform.

2.5.2. Activities for Certification

For schools to be successful in achieving the activities needed for certification, there is a yearly planner with guideline dates for task completion that the schools will use to keep on track. This also includes the accreditation visit. For example, the SLASF slideshows for the staff, team and youth leaders need to have been completed before the 2nd week of the school year. A designated training day takes place a week later. The purpose of this training day is to introduce the pilot schools to each other and the research team. The research team describes the whole year process evaluation and measurements taken throughout the year. There are co-design opportunities between the TY leaders and researchers to formulate the surveys used to collect data. The training day is not expected to run every year once feasibility is over. At this training day, two members of staff, the SLASF coordinator and another on the SLASF team take four student leaders to a training venue to learn about how to run the activities throughout the year. The website should also go live at the outset of the process. The website should encompass an easy to find link to the SLASF section of the site and there are the four core parts of the SLASF process; Physical Education; PA; Partnerships; and Active School Week.

- Another activity that the school needs to complete is the SLASF Awareness Week. This should be completed two weeks after the training day.
- School census questionnaire is deployed a week after the awareness week and this precedes the official launch of the SLASF process.
- During the launch, there would be a school wide tug of war (TOW) competition that is planned, promoted and organised by the SLASF committee.
- For the launch day the overall winning TOW team will compete against a staff team at a whole school event to launch the SLASF initiative.

A school census questionnaire was developed to help the SLASF team to identify their action plan. Core questions about PA opportunities, physical education, involvement in extra-curriculum activities and barriers to PA were included in an online survey. For a week after the awareness week, the survey is available for completion. All responses are anonymous and completed confidentially. Class teachers supervise and help answer any technical questions related to the completion of the survey. The data is stored on a secure server that is only accessible to the researchers. However, the overall results for each variable would be computed and provided for the school to carry out their own descriptive analyses with the TY group. The TY class can then produce meaningful findings from the survey to show the school through the notice board and used for one of the planned actions.

For the TOW event a free rope and a 2 1/2 h workshop will be provided for each school. This will enable TYs to coach and officiate TOW competitions and SLASF committee members that complete the course will receive a TOW Community Coach certificate upon completion. Each class in the school will be involved in this event with each having 3 TOW teams that compete against each other during tutor time or physical education class to decide what team will represent the class. Each class TOW team competes against the other classes in their year group during lunchtime to find the best TOW team for their year. Local role models can be invited to help launch the event by taking part in one of the TOW teams. This event should take place before the mid-autumn break.

After the mid-autumn break, the schools would have access to their school's results from the school questionnaire. The SLASF teams are given a month to review the results and start to design an SLASF action plan. At least three action points need to be agreed upon by the SLASF team. The proposed SLASF actions should be presented to the Principal for agreement. The agreed actions are then implemented in the second half of the school year. Towards the end of the year, the three agreed actions will be reviewed by the SLASF team members and presented to the school Principal during the last two weeks of the school year.

In addition, all students in the selected year group in the school will take part in a four weeks PA module delivered by the Social and Personal Health Education (SPHE) teachers. There would have to be a 'Did You Know?' campaign around the school that helps raise awareness about the benefits of PA for teenagers, in particular the positive impact that PA has upon focus, concentration and academic achievement. Another practical task for the SLASF team is to signpost an Active School WALKWAY. The walkway is a route that can be used by the students in the school during recess time or under teacher supervision for active learning activities, before/after tests or during free classes. SLASF, in partnership with Get Ireland Walking, designed Active School WALKWAY packs consisting of colourful outdoor all-weather sign post plaques which include orienteering symbols. One of the tasks that the SLASF TY class have to undertake is to map, measure and erect the walkway signposts to create a school walking route. A school WALKWAY Day where all classes get the opportunity to complete the walkway route with their teachers on a nominated school day needs to be agreed by school management. Then it is organised and promoted by the SLASF TY team. The organised walkway can be used as part of orienteering activities during timetabled physical education, as well as other school-based initiatives.

As the year ends, the school prepares for the accreditation visit for the certificate. A follow up visit takes place during the acquisition of the flag year. Prior to this, the school needs to organise a community mapping exercise and community events which should help with the design of the Active School Week (ASW) programme. The main aims of the ASW are to promote PA in a fun and inclusive way, as well as raising awareness about the availability and variety of PA opportunities for teenagers and their families in their local community. Throughout this week the school provides many and varied opportunities for staff and students to become more physically active throughout the school day.

2.5.3. Expected Outcomes Tables and Measures

According to their training resources, the programme aims to impact on a number of areas. However, to measure them all, multiple sources are required. A collection of survey instruments can be used to measure some of the outcomes, whereas some interviews can be used to evaluate other outcomes. In addition, the programme is year-long and a whole-school approach, hence site visits and checking on progress through logbook entries would be used to determine the processes carried out during the study. In Table 2, there is a list of the areas that SLASF aims to promote and some measures that can be used to test these outcomes.

Table 2. Aligning outcomes with measures.

SLASF Target Areas	Measures of Efficacy	Details
Physically educated	Self-efficacy in PA	Student survey
Physically active school community	Comprehensive Survey and focus groups	Survey item and discussions
Broad physical education	Whole-school survey and focus groups	List of physical education activities and discussions
Balanced physical education	Teacher scheme of work	Teacher records
More inclusiveness	Teacher scheme of work	Teacher records
Partnership with others to promote pa culture	TY logbook	Taster session from ASW
Active school week	TY logbook	Record of entries
Increased concentration	Harter scale	Student survey
Improved learning	Teachers perceptions	Student and teacher survey
Maintenance of discipline	Teacher records	Discipline records
Improved test results	Winter and summer test	Academic records
School enjoyment	Questionnaire	Student survey
Increase Daily PA	Accelerometers	Comprehensive Data
Reduced sitting time	Accelerometers	Comprehensive Data
Reduction in overweight and obesity	Self-report and anthropometric measures of height and weight	Comprehensive data

2.5.4. Questionnaires

There are two types of online surveys carried out throughout the year. The basic survey is completed by the entire school. This survey is anonymous and the focus is on PA participation and barriers to school related physical activities. This survey is a compulsory part of the SLASF process. Administration of the survey is decided by the school, with the intention to cover the entire school. Ideally, a census sweep of the school takes place at the same time. However, there may be some technical issues that may prevent this from happening. For example, schools may have a limited number of computers accessing the internet at any one time (bandwidth limits), may have a limited number of units to complete the survey (lack of tablets or computers) or could not get all the school to take part at the same time (timetabling issues). The results of the survey will be given back to the school for the purpose to plan specific school-based interventions. Therefore, it is important that the mode of data collection, analysis and reporting can be completed quickly and easily. Failing all technical capabilities to collect from an online platform, extra resources would be dedicated to ensure double coding from pen and paper surveys.

The second type of survey is a comprehensive survey, used for evaluating the feasibility of the study. The participants in this study input their user-ID so that the data can be linked from the beginning and end of the year long programme. Completion of the online survey takes place as one of the testing stations during the data collection visits. All the students have tablets or allocated to a school computer to complete the online survey. Details of the instruments are reported in Table 3.

Table 3. Battery of questionnaires.

Battery	Items	Response Scales	Psychometric Information
PA Screening measure	2 items on number of days in a week of at least 60 min of MVPA per day	0–7 days	Validity & Reliability [5,44]
PA opportunities	Modified items about local opportunities for PA to the context of schools instead of 'residential area'	5 point scale, 1 = disagree a lot, 5 = agree a lot	Original items used from an interview guide.
The exercise self-efficacy scale for adolescents	10 items on confidence to participate in a variety of conditions	11 point sliding scale, 0 = not at all confident, 10 = very confident	Nigg & Courneya, 1999 [45]
PA peer support scale	4 items on the frequency of peers influence for PA	0 = never, 5 = every day	Prochaska et al., 2002 [46]
PA, plans, expectancy and intention	Modified 3 items on the planning, expectancy and intention to do PA in the coming week	1 = unlikely, 8 = likely	Hagger et al., 2001 [47]
Readiness for behaviour change	Single item to determine which stage of the transtheoretical model in terms of PA	Select one item of each stage of the transtheoretical model	Lee et al., 2001 [48]
Perceived school performance	Single item about perceptions of teacher's evaluation of students' grade	Very good, good, average, below average	Felder-Puig et al., 2012 [49]
Perceived school performance	Two items about the students perception of their school grades	5 point scale, 1 = strongly disagree, 5 = strongly agree	Felder-Puig et al., 2012 [49]
Harter's Self-perception scale for adolescents	5 items from the scholastic competence subscale.	Polarised responding	Harter et al., 1982 [50]
Belonging in school	2 items on belonging to a school	1 = Strongly agree, 5 = strongly disagree	OECD
School satisfaction	How do you feel about school a present	1 = I like it a lot, 5 = I don't like it at all	HBSC since 2001
School effort	How pressured do you feel by the schoolwork you have to do	Not at all A little, Some, A lot	HBSC since 2001
Participation of organised activities	3 items about the student-led activities at school.	1 = Strongly agree, 5 = strongly disagree	HBSC in 2013/14
Kidscreen-27	Items on the physical and psychological well-being and the autonomy and parent relations	Not at all, Slightly, Moderately, Extremely	Ravens-Sieberer, et al., 2006 [51]

2.6. Process Evaluation

2.6.1. Logbook Activities

Each school is given a logbook to record their activities. This is used as part of the accreditation process and is used by the researchers to evaluate the processes that the school used. The logbook is mainly used by the SLASF team and the SLASF committees. Every week, the TY students have the opportunity to complete a small section in the diary to record what took place. The diary is linked to the school year and the expected timescale for carrying out specific activities. There is also a chart for the SLASF team to complete by recording the agreed actions to be carried out by the SLASF team. The team need to record the date of the agreed action, a short title for the action, the person(s) responsible, date of the action completed and a check box.

The TY team carries out a brief version of the System of Observing Play and Leisure Activity in Youth (SOPLAY) [52]. SOPLAY is a direct observation tool that is used by the TYs to assess PA levels within specific PA areas in the school. Due to resources, the full SOPLAY protocol had to be reduced down to three specific areas around the school. Furthermore, the TYs use tablets to video record the specific area and retrospectively carry out the observations. It is designed in this way because the technology is more readily available in schools than the time when SOPLAY was created by McKenzie and colleagues [52]. Through, observing the video recordings, the results can be verified so the validity of the results are stronger. Trained researchers with the SOPLAY counting system can verify the results from the TYs by matching the observation results. The videos can also be used as part of a TY class, where the students can get an understanding of ways to record the different intensities of PA. The SOPLAY exercise is carried out over six times throughout the school year. The assignment of the dates are researcher assigned days. The TYs are informed of the audit in the morning of the day the recording takes place. To reduce potential bias in the results, the TYs are reminded not to tell others that they are carrying out the observation. Observations take place twice during lunchtimes, one 10 min into the beginning and the second when there is 10 min left.

Another activity recorded in the logbook is the SLASF committee meetings. The logbook provides space for six meetings throughout the year. The meeting minutes include the people in attendance, the areas of discussion and the actions that were agreed. There is also space in the logbook has space for a list of agreed action created by the TY class during their timetabled class time. To encourage compliance, there is room for information such as the agreed action, the person responsible and the date for completion. In addition, there is room in the logbook for the TY team and coordinator to note activities that take place in a specific week. For each week, tasks that are suggested, such as the slide show, presentation of the action plan and so forth are available for the TY and coordinator to help remind to be on track.

2.6.2. Whole-School Surveys

There are three surveys to be carried out by all students in the school. The whole-school survey is part of the feasibility study and is carried out through an online survey platform. It is a mandatory action to be carried out by the school and is carried out during the first two months of the academic year. The school uses this information for creating and implementing three school specific action plans. Within this survey there are details of participation levels and barriers to taking part in physical education and extra curriculum activities. Both staff and students complete a second survey halfway through the process with items also related to process evaluation. Items will test implementation, fidelity and satisfaction of the tasks completed to date. The final whole-school survey has items related to process evaluation and is completed towards the end of the academic year but before the accreditation visit. The survey will also be held on an online survey platform. Due to the difficulties in getting whole-school engagement towards the end of the school year, the survey has pragmatic evaluation items whereby it can be completed on a mobile device such as a tablet or smart phone.

2.7. Sample Size

There are three schools that are part of the feasibility study. Unlike a sample size calculation, a justification is made for feasibility studies [53]. In Table 4, information about the size of the school, the type and the number of participants expected to complete the comprehensive arm of the study is presented.

According to the Department of Education and Skills school lists, School B is one of the largest secondary level in Ireland, with 1313 enrolled students. It is also a DEIS school. Approximately 10% of secondary level students attend a DEIS designated school. Moreover, there are known socioeconomic barriers towards PA [6], therefore it is necessary to carry out this feasibility in a DEIS school environment. School A is an all-girls school. Almost one in five schools in the country are all-girls' schools. There are many reports of girls having lower levels of PA than boys and therefore it is essential to include an all-girl's school. School C has a slightly fewer number of students than the national average of 999 students per school. Moreover, the ratio between girls and boys is slightly higher for girls (1:1.05), whereas the national average in mixed schools tends to have fewer girls than boys (1:0.87).

Table 4. Sample size descriptions.

School	Students	Girls	Boys	Teachers	DEIS	Comprehensive (N)
Intervention						
A	971	971	-	70	N	100
B	863	440	423	70	N	150
C	1313	664	649	120	Y	150
Control						
D	582	582	-	41	N	123
E	629	322	307	45	N	121
F	378	206	172	35	Y	88

2.8. Data Analyses

2.8.1. Quantitative Data

The data from the surveys are analysed through relevant statistical methods for the follow up data in this feasibility study. Compatible data between comprehensive and basic surveys can be used to determine the test-retest reliability of the items given that a smaller subsample of the entire school. As reliability is an important psychometric property for question items, this is carried out during the first phase of data collection.

Students take part in the comprehensive study have their measures taken two times during the academic year. The first time takes place in autumn 2018 and the second takes place six months later during the spring 2019. Accelerometer data are transferred through the ActivPal software based on 15sec epoch. The standardised cut-offs for different types of motion; sleep, standing, light, moderate and vigorous PA are then compared at an individual level from pre- and post-test time points. Similarly, the height, weight and grip strength data is compared between the time points and used to control the differences in accelerometer data. Comprehensive survey data is also analysed with differences in PA and school related factors.

Exploratory approaches include cross-sectional multivariate analyses of PA and school-related factors as independent variables and device-based PA and perceptions of PA opportunities as the dependent variables. Mixed models and multi-level regression analyses can be used on the data that has sufficient follow up data from the first time point. The multi-level approach takes into account between- and within- individual processes that explain variances in the outcome measures. Through this approach, it is possible to test the extent of PA (psychosocial variables) and school-related factors in relation to changes in PA levels and opportunities, at the same time to examine the individual versus the school factors that contribute to the outcome variables.

The follow-up data adds another level of analysis that can test the changes through the intervention. It makes it possible to examine, for example, the changes in PA levels across the schools from the beginning and the end of the study, while also taking into account changes in the psychosocial variables included in this study. The interactions between the contexts can confirm behavioural change theories by examining the mediating and moderation mechanisms in PA levels. The majority of the statistical analysis would be carried out using IBM SPSS.

2.8.2. Qualitative Data

The majority of the qualitative data comprises of focus group data. The way data is captured is a summary of individuals who collectively agree and discuss on the content [54]. Therefore, the first phase of analysis is to provide quantitative analysis of the subjects and the group types [55]. Focus groups can be useful to find a consensus on a phenomenon, as well as to engage with participants to discuss and share ideas that would otherwise be difficult to gather from one to one interviews [56]. In particular, the structural approach to children's group research can be used and transferred across to adolescents so that the students' voice to be heard [57]. Because the way a person in the focus group may consider a way to respond to the moderators' questions could differ from what other individuals may be thinking at the time, it is important to consider the way individuals respond, with whom and in what ways [55]. Transcriptions are matched with assistant moderator notes of verbal and non-verbal behaviours.

The data from one-to-one interviews is more straightforward. A semi-structure interview guide is used to direct the respondent to focus on the research questions and is used for further probing into these questions if the respondent needs to explain something further. Interviewees data are also merged with intonation coding to help reinforce the importance of non-verbal behaviour. The double coding from the transcription across the different qualitative approaches creates a rich source of data.

The combination of data is inserted into NVivo software for qualitative analysis. The metadata and types of data are used to create a rich data set. The data undergoes a thematic analysis as suggested by Lederman [58] by (1) identifying the big ideas, (2) creating units of data, (3) categorizing the units, (4) negotiating categories and (5) identifying themes and use of theory. The theories surrounding social-cognitive theories, including self-efficacy theory [29], self-determination theory [31] and competence motivation theory [50] are lens used in the final steps of the content analyses.

The data are collected through follow up measures throughout the year. The researchers incorporate verification checking at the beginning of each session to place a point where the respondents can focus on. In particular, we are interested in the processes of the intervention, as well as the potential transformation in beliefs, thoughts and actions over the course of the year. These steps are useful for designing the results in a way that allows for multi-method approach to the overall research questions.

2.8.3. Mixed Methods Analyses

Both quantitative and qualitative data can complement each other. We hope that the data that derives from both methods of inquiry can be partly explained through the literature to date and other types of data that is collected. To return to the points of evaluation of the feasibility study, there are various numbers of expected outcomes that the school is expected to achieve and they are measured directed through particular sources (Table 2). For example, the expected outcome of a broad physical education curriculum is measured through the whole school survey on participation of various physical education activities. The data taken from the beginning of the year gives insight to the types of activities that the students reported to have attended in the past 12 months. Through data collection across all year groups, the survey data can be used to determine how broad the physical education programme actually is. The post-test survey would give an indication of the extent of the physical education programme. However, reliance solely on this measure may be limited to the actual item that is included in the survey [59]. Therefore, combining the data from focus groups by the students and staff at the school can give more details about what was popular, who experienced the changes and the mechanisms in place to make the broader physical education opportunities. Therefore, the focus on the results are on the processes of creating the change, thus allowing further insight into the behavioural change techniques used to facilitate such changes.

The SLASF log data contains both quantitative and qualitative data and can be analysed for the percent of completion towards the SLASF. Actions in relation to SLASF throughout the year form descriptive feasibility analyses. Differences in the PA audit across the year are analysed through descriptive statistics over time. In combination with the logbook of actions and the results of the PA audit more details about the feasibility of schools' actions from the TY class can be determined in relation to desired outcomes.

2.9. Availability of Data and Materials

After completion of the study, data will be stored at the University of Limerick's Data archive without potential identifiers and request for data can be made through the study's principal investigator (Last author). All supplementary materials for the SLASF programme including the resource pack, template logbook and accompanying resources will be available at https://osf.io/frx6t/.

2.10. Ethics Approval and Consent to Participate

The study follows the principles of the Declaration of Helsinki. The study protocol has been approved by the research ethics committee of the Faculty of Education and Health Sciences, University of Limerick (ref no. 2018/10/18_EHS). Written informed consent will be sought from participating teachers, students and students' guardians. All participants have permission to withdraw from the study at any time and data deleted if collected. In cases of important protocol changes, requests from the ethical committee will be sought for. Trial Registration: https://osf.io/keubz/register/5771ca429ad5a1020de2872e; Registered 24th September 2018; Clinical Trial Registration: NCT03847831.

3. Discussion

In this year-long feasibility study of the SLASF, a mixed-method approach is used to give recommendation to stop, revise or conduct a randomised control trial. The whole-school approach requires multiple stakeholders, primarily the students in secondary level schools, the TY students, the SLASF staff and its committee, as well as the management. The theories used in this paper are based on social cognitive theories and stages of change model [29,31,50].

Whole-school based interventions in the promotion of PA have been increasing [11,19] although the inception of the SLASF in the secondary level schools is more complicated than primary level schools. The diversity of foci at secondary level schools brings challenges towards a uniform and national programme. This is evident to date, whereby 29% of primary schools are ASF schools, whereas less than 5% of secondary level schools have this status. Therefore, a feasibility study is needed to test the readiness prior to national roll-out.

The results from this study would be used to help inform the development of the SLASF and report the experiences of the schools in the feasibility study. Secondary outcomes from the measures carried out in the study may lead to improved understanding of the mechanisms of the promotion of PA. Moreover, the direct mapping of the stated goals of the SLASF with measures would provide evidence. Future iterations of the SLASF may include opt in by the students to take part in the SLASF TY programme, thus providing a mixture of students who are active and inactive.

The challenges to this programme include the fidelity of the year-long programme. Schools are dynamic systems all with different characteristics based on the people who attend it. Challenging aspects could include issues arising from the coordination of the staff and pupils to carry out the tasks. There may be other activities that take place in the school, which reduce the efforts needed to run the programme or conversely, highly engagement that roles are dispersed more than previously planned. Monitoring of fidelity and carrying out process evaluations would help inform the way the programme is run.

This feasibility study is novel in design in that it a whole-school approach to the promotion of physical activity among adolescents who are empowered to organize activities over the course of the year. School management also receive an incentive by striving towards the goal and recognition of

J. Funct. Morphol. Kinesiol. **2019**, *4*, 16

an Active School Flag. Successful piloting of the SLASF can lead to upscaling to all secondary level schools around the Republic of Ireland due to the programme endorsement by the Department of Education and Skills. Testing of the programme can be part of large scale RCT that would fit under the Healthy Ireland Demonstration Project.

Author Contributions: K.W.N. drafted the manuscript. All authors were responsible for writing part of the manuscript and critically revising the complete manuscript. F.M. contributed to the background and concept of the study. K.C. contributed to the design of the programme. D.O. contributed to the study design. C.W. is the principal investigator and contributed to the concept and design of the study. All authors approved the final manuscript.

Funding: The feasibility study is funded by Mayo Education Centre, Healthy Ireland and St. Vincent's Foundation.

Acknowledgments: K.W.N., F.M., D.O. and C.W. are researchers who have remained independent in the design of the SLASF programme. K.C. is a member of the ASF steering committee and designed the SLASF programme. K.C.'s involvement was to ensure all the aspects of this protocol are correct. K.C. has no involvement with carrying out the research, either in data collection or analyses.

Conflicts of Interest: K.C. is employed by the Mayo Education Centre although K.C. is not involved in carrying out the research. All other authors declare that they have no competing interests.

References

1. Patton, G.C.; Sawyer, S.M.; Santelli, J.S.; Ross, D.A.; Afifi, R.; Allen, N.B.; Arora, M.; Azzopardi, P.; Baldwin, W.; Bonell, C.; et al. Our future: A Lancet commission on adolescent health and wellbeing. *Lancet* **2016**, *387*, 2423–2478. [CrossRef]
2. Telama, R. Tracking of physical activity from childhood to adulthood: A review. *Obes. Facts* **2009**, *2*, 187–195. [CrossRef] [PubMed]
3. Woods, C.B.; Tannerhill, D.; Quinlan, A.; Moyna, N.; Walsh, J. *The Children's Sport Participation and Physical Activity Study (CSPPA)*; Irish Sports Council: Dublin, Ireland, 2010.
4. Dumith, S.C.; Gigante, D.P.; Domingues, M.R.; Kohl, H.W. Physical activity change during adolescence: A systematic review and a pooled analysis. *Int. J. Epidemiol.* **2011**, *40*, 685–698. [CrossRef] [PubMed]
5. Hardie Murphy, M.; Rowe, D.A.; Woods, C.B. Impact of physical activity domain on subsequent activity in youth: A 5-year longitudinal study. *J. Sports Sci.* **2017**, *35*, 262–268. [CrossRef]
6. Inchley, J.; Currie, D.; Young, T.; Samdal, O.; Torsheim, T.; Augustson, L.; Mathison, F.; Aleman-Diaz, A.; Molcho, M.; Weber, M.; Barnekow, V. *Growing Up Unequal: Gender and Socioeconomic Differences in Young People's Health and Well-Being. Health Behaviour in School-Aged Children (HBSC) Study: International Report from the 2013/2014 Survey*; Report No.: Health Policy for Children and Adolescents, No.7; WHO Regional Office for Europe: Copenhagen, Denmark, 2016.
7. Schilling, J.M.; GilesCorti, B.; Sallis, J.F. Connecting active living research and public policy: Transdisciplinary research and policy interventions to increase physical activity. *J. Public Health Policy* **2009**, *30* (Suppl. 1), S1–S15. [CrossRef] [PubMed]
8. Masters, R.; Anwar, E.; Collins, B.; Cookson, R.; Capewell, S. Return on investment of public health interventions: A systematic review. *J. Epidemiol. Community Health* **2017**, *71*, 827–834. [CrossRef]
9. Love, R.; Adams, J.; van Sluijs, E.M.F. Are school-based physical activity interventions effective and equitable? A meta-analysis of cluster randomized controlled trials with accelerometer-assessed activity. *Obes. Rev.* **2019**. [CrossRef]
10. Pate, R.R.; Dowda, M. Raising an Active and Healthy Generation: A Comprehensive Public Health Initiative. *Exerc. Sport Sci. Rev.* **2019**, *47*, 3–14. [CrossRef]
11. Haapala, H.L.; Hirvensalo, M.H.; Laine, K.; Laakso, L.; Hakonen, H.; Kankaanpää, A.; Lintunen, T.; Tammelin, T.H. Recess physical activity and school-related social factors in Finnish primary and lower secondary schools: Cross-sectional associations. *BMC Public Health* **2014**, *14*, 1114. [CrossRef]
12. Carlin, A.; Murphy, M.H.; Nevill, A.; Gallagher, A.M. Effects of a peer-led Walking in ScHools intervention (the WISH study) on physical activity levels of adolescent girls: A cluster randomised pilot study. *Trials* **2018**, *19*, 31. [CrossRef]

13. Owen, M.B.; Kerner, C.; Taylor, S.L.; Noonan, R.J.; Newson, L.; Kosteli, M.C.; Curry, W.B.; Fairclough, S.J. The Feasibility of a Novel School Peer-Led Mentoring Model to Improve the Physical Activity Levels and Sedentary Time of Adolescent Girls: The Girls Peer Activity (G-PACT) Project. *Children* **2018**, *5*, 67. [CrossRef]

14. Sebire, S.J.; Jago, R.; Banfield, K.; Edwards, M.J.; Campbell, R.; Kipping, R.; Blair, P.S.; Kadir, B.; Garfield, K.; Matthews, J.; et al. Results of a feasibility cluster randomised controlled trial of a peer-led school-based intervention to increase the physical activity of adolescent girls (PLAN-A). *Int. J. Behav. Nutr. Phys. Act.* **2018**, *15*, 50. [CrossRef] [PubMed]

15. Lubans, D.; Morgan, P. Impact of an extra-curricular school sport programme on determinants of objectively measured physical activity among adolescents. *Health Educ. J.* **2008**, *67*, 305–320. [CrossRef]

16. Lubans, D.R.; Morgan, P.J.; Aguiar, E.J.; Callister, R. Randomized controlled trial of the Physical Activity Leaders (PALs) program for adolescent boys from disadvantaged secondary schools. *Prev. Med.* **2011**, *52*, 239–246. [CrossRef]

17. Smith, J.J.; Morgan, P.J.; Plotnikoff, R.C.; Stodden, D.F.; Lubans, D.R. Mediating effects of resistance training skill competency on health-related fitness and physical activity: The ATLAS cluster randomised controlled trial. *J. Sports Sci.* **2016**, *34*, 772–779. [CrossRef]

18. Dobbins, M.; Husson, H.; DeCorby, K.; LaRocca, R.L. School-based physical activity programs for promoting physical activity and fitness in children and adolescents aged 6 to 18. *Cochrane Database Syst. Rev.* **2013**, *2*. [CrossRef]

19. McMullen, J.; Ní Chróinín, D.; Tammelin, T.; Pogorzelska, M.; van der Mars, H. International Approaches to Whole-of-School Physical Activity Promotion. *Quest* **2015**, *67*, 384–399. [CrossRef]

20. Davison, K.K.; Jago, R. Change in parent and peer support across ages 9 to 15 yr and adolescent girls' physical activity. *Med. Sci. Sports Exerc.* **2009**, *41*, 1816–1825. [CrossRef]

21. Fitzgerald, A.; Fitzgerald, N.; Aherne, C. Do peers matter? A review of peer and/or friends' influence on physical activity among American adolescents. *J. Adolesc.* **2012**, *35*, 941–958. [CrossRef]

22. Jenkinson, K.A.; Benson, A.C. Barriers to Providing Physical Education and Physical Activity in Victorian State Secondary Schools. *Aust. J. Teach. Educ.* **2010**, *35*, 1–17. [CrossRef]

23. Clerkin, A. Personal development in secondary education: The Irish transition year. *Educ. Policy Anal. Arch.* **2012**, *20*. [CrossRef]

24. Jeffers, G. The Transition Year programme in Ireland. Embracing and resisting a curriculum innovation. *Curric. J.* **2011**, *22*, 61–76. [CrossRef]

25. Kelleher, C.; Kelly, D.; Finnegan, O.; Kerley, M.; Doherty, K.; Gilroy, I.; Conlon, G.; Fitzpatrick, P.; Daly, L. Gender and content influence second-level students' expectations of health education seminars provided in a health promoting hopital setting. *Clin. Health Promot.* **2014**, *4*, 5–11.

26. Hayes, S. A Critical Examination and Evaluation of the Place of Science in the Irish Transition Year. Ph.D. Thesis, University of Limerick, Limerick, Ireland, 2011.

27. Plotnikoff, R.C.; Costigan, S.A.; Karunamuni, N.; Lubans, D.R. Social cognitive theories used to explain physical activity behavior in adolescents: A systematic review and meta-analysis. *Prev. Med.* **2013**, *56*, 245–253. [CrossRef] [PubMed]

28. Davis, R.; Campbell, R.; Hildon, Z.; Hobbs, L.; Michie, S. Theories of behaviour and behaviour change across the social and behavioural sciences: A scoping review. *Health Psychol. Rev.* **2015**, *9*, 323–344. [CrossRef]

29. Bandura, A. Self-efficacy: Toward a unifying theory of behavioral change. *Psychol. Rev.* **1977**, *84*, 191–215. [CrossRef] [PubMed]

30. Martin, J.J.; Kulinna, P.H. A Social Cognitive Perspective of Physical-Activity-Related Behavior in Physical Education. *J. Teach. Phys. Educ.* **2005**, *24*, 265–281. [CrossRef]

31. Deci, E.L.; Ryan, R.M. *Intrinsic Motivation and Self-Determination in Human Behaviour*; Plenum Press: New York, NY, USA, 1985.

32. Hagger, M.S.; Chatzisarantis, N.L.D.; Culverhouse, T.; Biddle, S.J.H. The Processes by Which Perceived Autonomy Support in Physical Education Promotes Leisure-Time Physical Activity Intentions and Behavior: A Trans-Contextual Model. *J. Educ. Psychol.* **2003**, *95*, 784–795. [CrossRef]

33. Hagger, M.S.; Chatzisarantis, N.L.D.; Hein, V.; Soos, I.; Karsai, I.; Lintunen, T.; Leemans, S. Teacher, peer and parent autonomy support in physical education and leisure-time physical activity: A trans-contextual model of motivation in four nations. *Psychol. Health* **2009**, *24*, 689–711. [CrossRef] [PubMed]

34. Mameli, C.; Molinari, L.; Passini, S. Agency and responsibility in adolescent students: A challenge for the societies of tomorrow. *Br. J. Educ. Psychol.* **2019**, *89*, 41–56. [CrossRef]

35. McNeely, C.; Falci, C. School Connectedness and the Transition into and Out of Health-Risk Behavior Among Adolescents: A Comparison of Social Belonging and Teacher Support. *J. Sch. Health* **2004**, *74*, 284–292. [CrossRef]

36. Dowd, A.J.; Chen, M.Y.; Jung, M.E.; Beauchamp, M.R. "Go Girls!" psychological and behavioral outcomes associated with a group-based healthy lifestyle program for adolescent girls. *Transl. Behav. Med.* **2015**, *5*, 77–86. [CrossRef]

37. Prochaska, J.O.; DiClemente, C.C. Stages and processes of self-change of smoking: Toward an integrative model of change. *J. Consult. Clin. Psychol.* **1983**, *51*, 390–395. [CrossRef]

38. De Bourdeaudhuij, I.; Philippaerts, R.; Crombez, G.; Matton, L.; Wijndaele, K.; Balduck, A.; Lefevre, J. Stages of change for physical activity in a community sample of adolescents. *Health Educ. Res.* **2005**, *20*, 357–366. [CrossRef]

39. Eldridge, S.M.; Lancaster, G.A.; Campbell, M.J.; Thabane, L.; Hopewell, S.; Coleman, C.L.; Bond, C.M. Defining Feasibility and Pilot Studies in Preparation for Randomised Controlled Trials: Development of a Conceptual Framework. *PLoS ONE* **2016**, *11*, e0150205. [CrossRef]

40. Bowen, D.J.; Kreuter, M.; Spring, B.; Cofta-Woerpel, L.; Linnan, L.; Weiner, D.; Bakken, S.; Kaplan, C.P.; Squiers, L.; Fabrizio, C.; et al. How We Design Feasibility Studies. *Am. J. Prev. Med.* **2009**, *36*, 452–457. [CrossRef]

41. Thabane, L.; Ma, J.; Chu, R.; Cheng, J.; Ismaila, A.; Rios, L.P.; Robson, R.; Thabane, M.; Giangregorio, L.; Goldsmith, C.H. A tutorial on pilot studies: The what, why and how. *BMC Med. Res. Methodol.* **2010**, *10*, 1. [CrossRef]

42. Ferguson, C.J.; Heene, M. A Vast Graveyard of Undead Theories: Publication Bias and Psychological Science's Aversion to the Null. *Perspect. Psychol. Sci.* **2012**, *7*, 555–561. [CrossRef]

43. Rosenbaum, P.; Gorter, J.W. The 'F-words' in childhood disability: I swear this is how we should think! *Child Care Health Dev.* **2012**, *38*, 457–463. [CrossRef]

44. Ng, K.; Hämylä, R.; Tynjälä, J.; Villberg, J.; Tammelin, T.; Kannas, L.; Kokko, S. Test-retest reliability of adolescents' self-reported physical activity item in two consecutive surveys. *Arch. Public Health* **2019**, *77*, 9. [CrossRef] [PubMed]

45. Nigg, C.R.; Courneya, K.S. Transtheoretical model: Examining adolescent exercise behavior. *J. Adoles. Health* **1998**, *22*, 214–224. [CrossRef]

46. Prochaska, J.J.; Rodgers, M.W.; Sallis, J.F. Association of Parent and Peer Support with Adolescent Physical Activity. *Res. Q. Exerc. Sport* **2002**, *73*, 206–2010. [CrossRef] [PubMed]

47. Hagger, M.S.; Chatzisarantis, N.L.D.; Biddle, S.J.H. The influence of self-efficacy and past behaviour on the physical activity intentions of young people. *J. Sports Sci.* **2001**, *19*, 711–725. [CrossRef] [PubMed]

48. Lee, R.E.; Nigg, C.R.; Diclemente, C.C.; Courneya, K.S. Validating Motivational Readiness for Exercise Behavior with Adolescents. *Res. Q. Exerc. Sport* **2001**, *72*, 401–410. [CrossRef] [PubMed]

49. Felder-Puig, R.; Griebler, R.; Samdal, O.; King, M.A.; Freeman, J.G.; Duer, W. Does the School Performance Variable Used in the International Health Behavior in School-Aged Children (HBSC) Study Reflect Students' School Grades? *J. Sch. Health* **2012**, *82*, 404–409. [CrossRef] [PubMed]

50. Harter, S. The Perceived Competence Scale for Children. *Child Dev.* **1982**, *53*, 87–97. [CrossRef]

51. Ravens-Sieberer, U.; KIDSCREEN Group Europe. *The KIDSCREEN Questionnaires. Quality of Life Questionnaires for Children and Adolescents—Handbook*; Papst Science Publisher: Lengerich, Germany, 2006.

52. McKenzie, T.L.; Marshall, S.J.; Sallis, J.F.; Conway, T.L. Leisure-time physical activity in school environments: An observational study using SOPLAY. *Prev. Med.* **2000**, *30*, 70–77. [CrossRef]

53. Lancaster, G.A. Pilot and feasibility studies come of age! *Pilot Feasibility Stud.* **2015**, *1*, 1. [CrossRef] [PubMed]

54. Krueger, R.A. *Developing Questions for Focus Groups*; Sage: Thousand Oaks, CA, USA, 1998.

55. Vaughn, S.; Schumm, J.S.; Sinagub, J. *Focus Group Interviews in Education and Psychology*; Sage Research Methods: Thousand Oaks, CA, USA, 2018.

56. Hollander, J.A. The social contexts of focus groups. *J. Contemp Ethnogr.* **2004**, *33*, 602–637. [CrossRef]

57. McDonald, W.J.; Topper, G.E. Focus group research with children: A structural approach. *Appl. Mark. Res.* **1988**, *28*, 3–11.

58. Lederman, L.C. Assessing educational effectiveness: The focus group interview as a technique for data collection. *Commun. Educ.* **1990**, *39*, 117–127. [CrossRef]
59. Moran, A.P.; Matthews, J.J.; Kirby, K. Whatever happened to the third paradigm? Exploring mixed methods research designs in sport and exercise psychology. *Qual. Res. Sport Exerc. Health* **2011**, *3*, 362–369. [CrossRef]

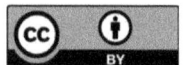

MDPI

St. Alban-Anlage 66

4052 Basel

Switzerland

Tel. +41 61 683 77 34

Fax +41 61 302 89 18

www.mdpi.com

Journal of Functional Morphology and Kinesiology Editorial Office

E-mail: jfmk@mdpi.com

www.mdpi.com/journal/jfmk

www.ingramcontent.com/pod-product-compliance
Lightning Source LLC
Chambersburg PA
CBHW041140120626
46547CB00020B/3062